ACOMPLIA
and
Your Hungry Brain

WHAT'S NEW IN WEIGHT-LOSS DRUGS

Kim Walker
Michael G. Walker PhD.

CURIOUS PRESS

2   ACOMPLIA AND YOUR HUNGRY BRAIN

Copyright © 2008 by Kim Walker and Michael G. Walker

All rights reserved.

No part of this book may be reproduced or transmitted in any form or by any means without written permission from the authors. Address inquiries to: permissions@curiouspress.com

This publication is designed to provide accurate and authoritative information but it is sold with the understanding that the publisher does not offer medical advice or other professional services.

Library of Congress Control Number: 2008901715
Includes Index

ISBN: 978-0-9802205-0-6

Curious Press
Los Altos, CA
USA

To the fire of my loins

...just as requested.

Acknowledgements

There is no substitute for being in the right place at the right time. The Stanford University School of Medicine is known as a leading institution of research and learning. For us, it is also a place of wonder and delight.

To colleagues and students alike, thank you for your inspiration and constant curiosity.

To our editor, Cindy Mark, we offer our thanks.

ACOMPLIA AND YOUR HUNGRY BRAIN

Contents

Introduction 9

Part One - The Big Picture

Acomplia - What is it? 15

    The Cannabis Connection 19

    Of Chemicals and Calories 23

Acomplia – Who Needs It? 29

Acomplia - Does It Work? 43

Part Two - The Usual Suspects

Dopamine - Signals of Desire 57

Cannabinoids - Old Dog, New Tricks 63

Opioids - Resistance is Futile 69

Cravings - Addiction Lite. 75

Melanocortins - Secret Ally. 81

Part Three - The Trials of Acomplia

Clinical Trials - Music To Our Ears 89

Side Effects - The Placebo Factor 95

Your Portrait - Painting by Numbers 101

Acomplia – Is It For You? 107

    Is Acomplia Safe? 109

    Is Acomplia Worth the Risks? 110

Acomplia and Diabetes 113

Part Four - Future Considerations

Alcohol - Rats That Drink and Drive 121

Nicotine - Furry Quitters 131

Drugs - No Rodent Left Behind. 139

Acomplia - Innovation In Research. 145

Acomplia - Future Treatments. 151

Final Note. 159

    Index 161

    References 167

    The Authors 176

WHAT'S NEW IN WEIGHT-LOSS DRUGS 7

8   ACOMPLIA AND YOUR HUNGRY BRAIN

*"Be careful of reading health books,
you might die of a misprint."*
~ Mark Twain

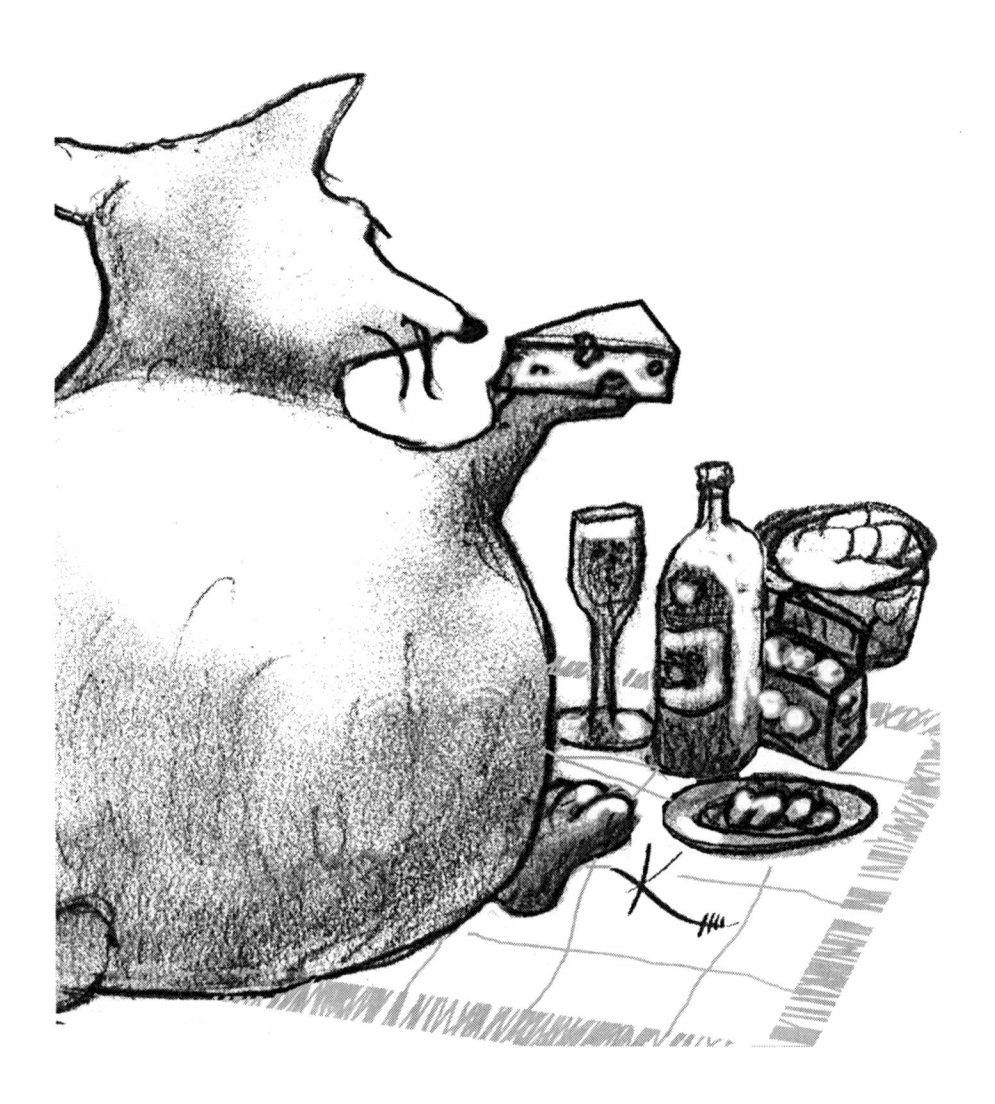

Introduction

Your brain is hungry. It uses more energy than any other organ in your body. Although it makes up as little as 2% of your body weight it uses as much as 20% of your total energy intake. The source of that energy is food and your brain never lets you forget it.

Sex, pain and fear occasionally drive your actions, but hunger is a constant master whether you realize it or not. Your brain controls the production of certain hormones to motivate your search for food and to reward you for feeding. Hunger is a powerful survival mechanism.

Even after eating, your brain is gearing up for the next meal. Chemical signals tell your brain the moment your stomach is empty; they report how much energy your liver has produced; they sound an alarm when energy levels drop. If you miss a meal, your brain takes steps to protect itself.

Hunger is the brain's way of getting your attention. If that doesn't work, it will start to restrict services: cutting back on your fine motor control, reducing your ability to concentrate and generally interfering with what you are doing until food arrives.

Your brain won't tap into that spare tire you carry around your middle until it has to – that's the emergency back-up. Instead, your brain systematically stores excess energy as fat as if it doesn't know what else to do. Over time, that extra fat takes on a life of its own, changing both your body and your mind.

Acomplia is a new drug that works directly on your brain by binding to the same sites that are stimulated by smoking marijuana. Around the world, Acomplia is recognized as an effective treatment for many over-weight patients, but if you live in America, the heaviest nation on earth, Acomplia is unavailable because it is not an approved weight-loss medication.

WHAT'S NEW IN WEIGHT-LOSS DRUGS

Acomplia is a man-made molecule that turns off cravings deep within your brain. Acomplia could help you lose weight; reduce your waist size; improve your cholesterol levels; lower your triglycerides and blood sugars; and generally reduce your risk of heart disease, diabetes and related cancers. It might help you quit smoking and avoid weight gain afterwards.

Here is the story of this amazing discovery that is changing the way we think about food addiction, the nature of weight gain and the intricate workings of the human brain.

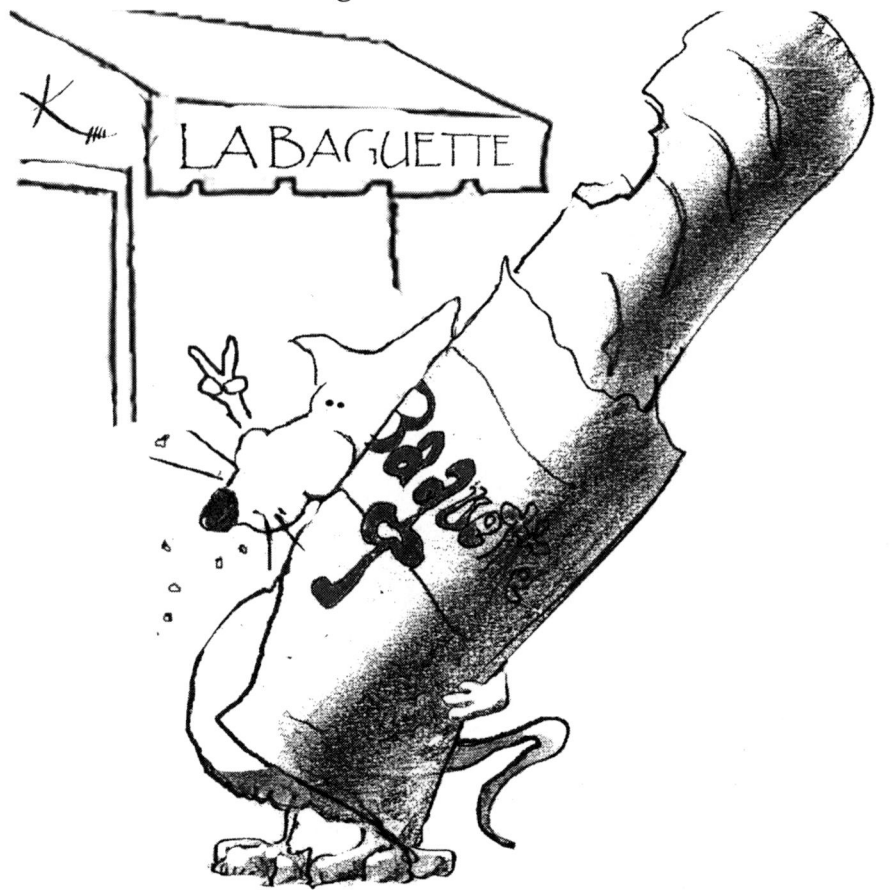

Flour Power

Part One

The Big Picture

14   ACOMPLIA AND YOUR HUNGRY BRAIN

*"It's all right letting yourself go,
as long as you can get yourself back."
~ Mick Jagger*

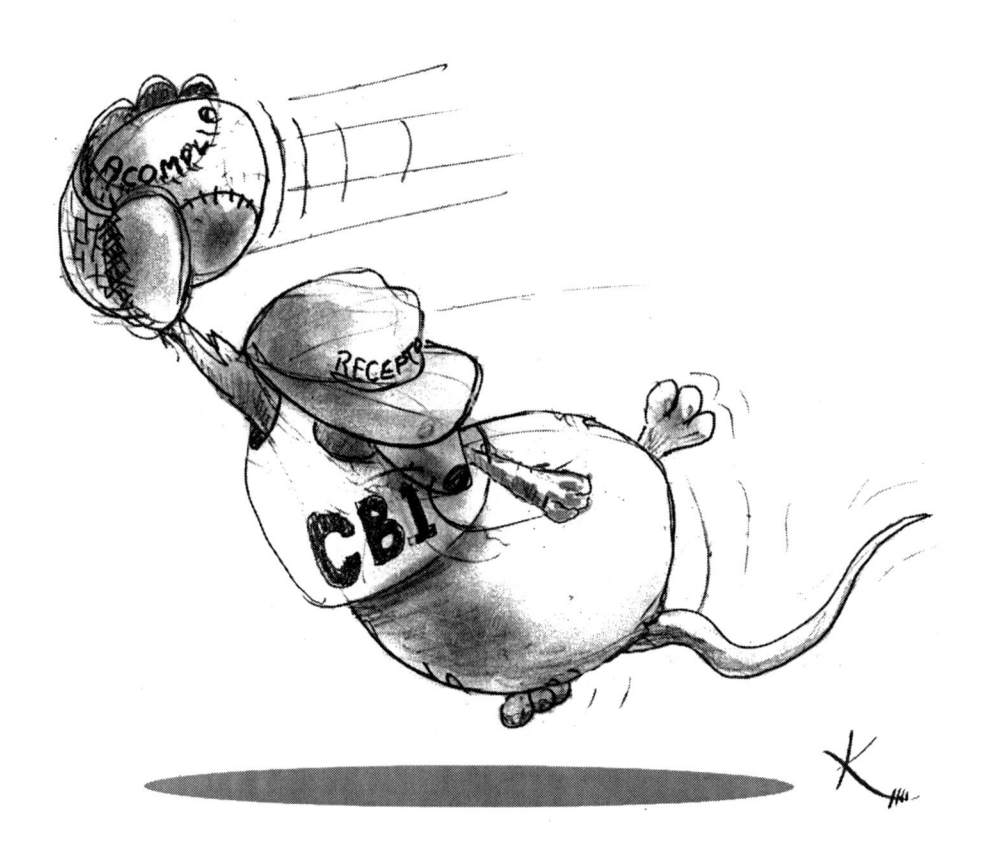

Acomplia - What is it?

Take a deep breath. Go ahead. Take a deep breath right now. Feel your lungs fill with air. Now exhale and hold your breath as oxygen is transferred from your lungs to your blood stream.

When you think about it, breathing usually occurs automatically without any conscious input from you. That's because receptors in your lungs signal your brain when it's time to take another breath. Your brain relies on that feedback to gauge the amount of oxygen available to your system.

Right about now, your brain is receiving signals warning of oxygen depletion in your lungs. Already you have an urge to breathe in because your brain is sending increasingly frantic signals down your phrenic nerve to your diaphragm, ordering it to contract. The longer you hold your breath, the more anxious you feel.

Now breathe normally again. You should feel a calming sense of relief as oxygen-rich air flows into your lungs? That's your reward for good behavior. You could consciously hold your breath for a minute or two, maybe longer, but eventually you will take a breath - whether you want to or not.

The idea that it might be fun to stop breathing for awhile originates in your forebrain where thoughts and decisions are made. Other parts of your brain are not so adventurous so no matter how hard you try to resist, sooner or later your so-called primitive brain, takes control and forces you to breathe again.

Obviously you need oxygen to stay conscious and alive. You also need food energy for the same reasons. Your brain monitors and regulates the energy needs of every cell in your body by receiving and sending signals over various nerve pathways to maintain homeostasis, the balance of life.

When cells need food, find food or consume it, they pass the information along by means of messenger molecules that dock with receptors on the surface of your brain the way a baseball fits into a catcher's glove.

Now imagine trying to catch a baseball when you have a grapefruit glued inside your mitt. It's not going to happen, is it? Acomplia is like that grapefruit. It is a small molecule that fits into your hunger receptors so perfectly that it blocks incoming signals, and prevents information from reaching your brain.

That sounds extreme, but it happens all the time. Receptors turn off and on regularly. At this moment, you have messenger molecules called hormones circulating through your body turning off certain receptors wherever they find them.

You also have hormones that turn receptors on. All your senses rely on active receptors to keep you in touch with the world around you. Molecules in your environment engage receptors in your ears, your eyes, in your mouth or up your nose to stimulate the secretion of hormones that carry information to receptors on the surface of your brain cells.

In contrast, you are unaware of receptors that monitor oxygen levels in your lungs, the presence of foreign bacteria on your skin or the amount of sugar in your blood. Receptors in your liver and other organs, even on your muscle and fat cells, trigger hormone release to send signals concerning your internal environment.

When certain receptors tell your brain that it is time to eat, you start to get hungry. You can deliberately refuse to eat just as you can stop breathing for awhile, but your hungry brain is more powerful than your thinking brain and it usually prevails.

If the receptors that stimulate appetite get over-excited they send unnecessary hunger signals to your brain. You may not be aware of it at first, but your body and your mind are mobilizing to search for food you don't really need. Acomplia can prevent that from happening.

18   ACOMPLIA AND YOUR HUNGRY BRAIN

"The saddest aspect of life right now is that science gathers knowledge faster than society gathers wisdom."
~ Isaac Asimov

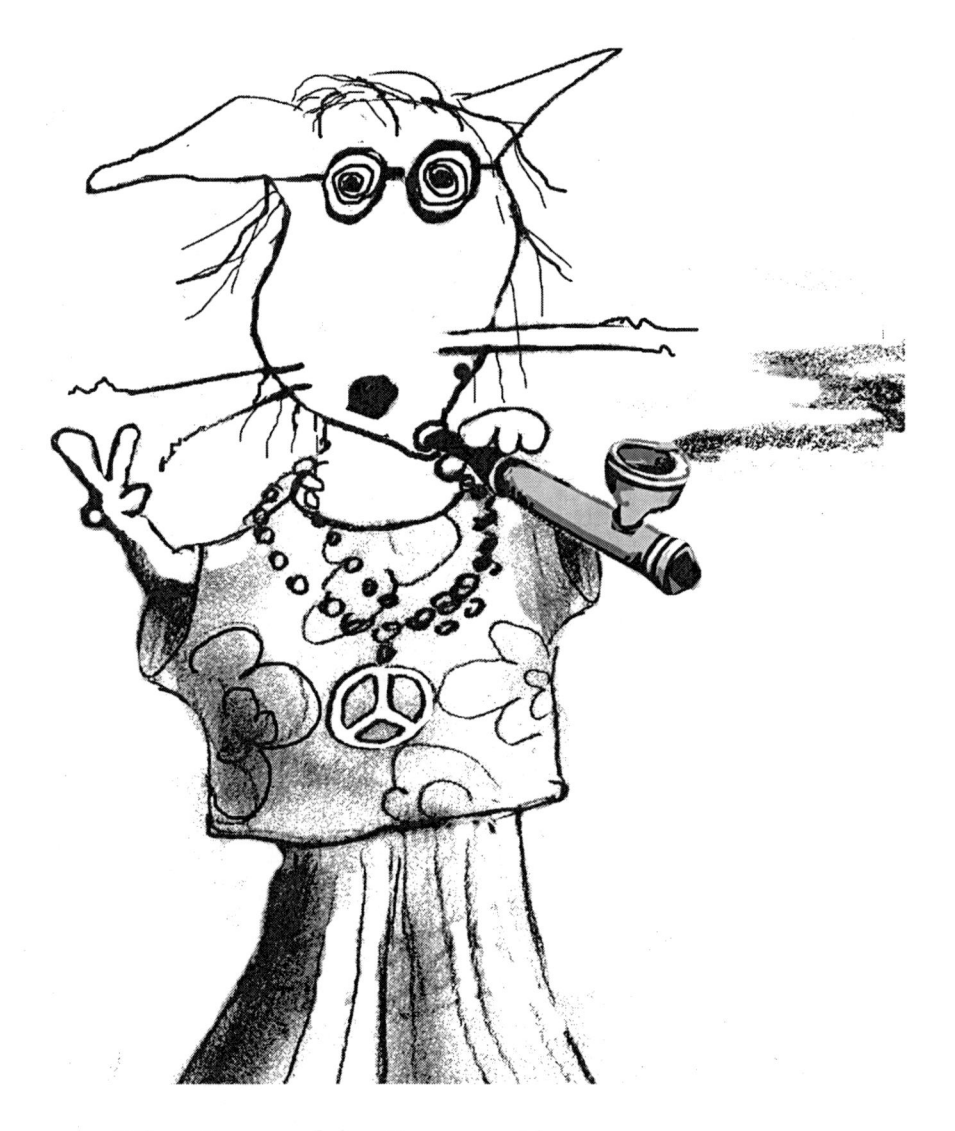

The Cannabis Connection

If you had discovered receptors that caused hunger, you might have called them cheesecake receptors, but somebody beat you to it. Today they are known as cannabinoid receptors because the scientists who found them were far more interested in cannabis than cheesecake.

Cannabis, better known as marijuana, was the recreational drug of choice during the 60's because of its pleasant, intoxicating effect - so I am told. It contains a psychoactive ingredient called THC (short for 9-tetrahydrocannabinol) that causes a 'high' or 'alternative consciousness' depending on who you talk to.

People under the influence of THC report that, apart from feeling really, really good, they feel really, really hungry. As side effects go, a case of the munchies seems harmless enough. More troubling is evidence that THC is responsible for selective memory loss. As the saying goes, if you remember the 60s, you weren't really there.

For some time, biochemists suspected that cannabis caused hunger by binding to receptors in the brain, but they were unable to prove it until 1984 when the existence of cannabinoid receptors was finally confirmed.

Not only did THC stimulate cannabinoid receptors sufficiently to induce hunger, constant stimulation led to overeating. More recent experiments suggest that over-active cannabinoid receptors also contribute to fat production.

THC is a plant product that does not occur naturally in humans or other mammals so obviously you must have something inside you similar to THC that whets your appetite.

In 1992, Drs. Hanus and Devane isolated a molecule that mimics THC.[2] It binds to cannabinoid receptors and stimulates the appetite and, like THC, it induces a sense of well being so they named it anandamide after the Sanskrit word *ananda*, meaning bliss.

WHAT'S NEW IN WEIGHT-LOSS DRUGS 21

Anandamide, the bliss molecule, is less powerful than THC and tends to break down quickly, yet it has an extraordinary effect on your behavior because it does something that only a few molecules can do - it crosses the blood-brain-barrier with ease.

You have a fatty membrane that protects your brain from direct contact with your blood stream. It is strong yet flexible protective shield that is usually difficult to penetrate, but Anandamide is equipped with a fatty protein on the tip of its tail that allows it to gain entry and wriggle through.

Anandamide has access to different parts of your brain where it affects signaling in a variety of ways. It also binds to opioid receptors to bring pleasure and pain relief. As both a cannabinoid and an opioid, anandamide reminds you when to eat and rewards you with pleasure when you do.

*"What some call health,
if purchased by the perpetual anxiety about diet,
isn't much better than tedious disease."
~ George Dennison Prentice (1860)*

To each his own.

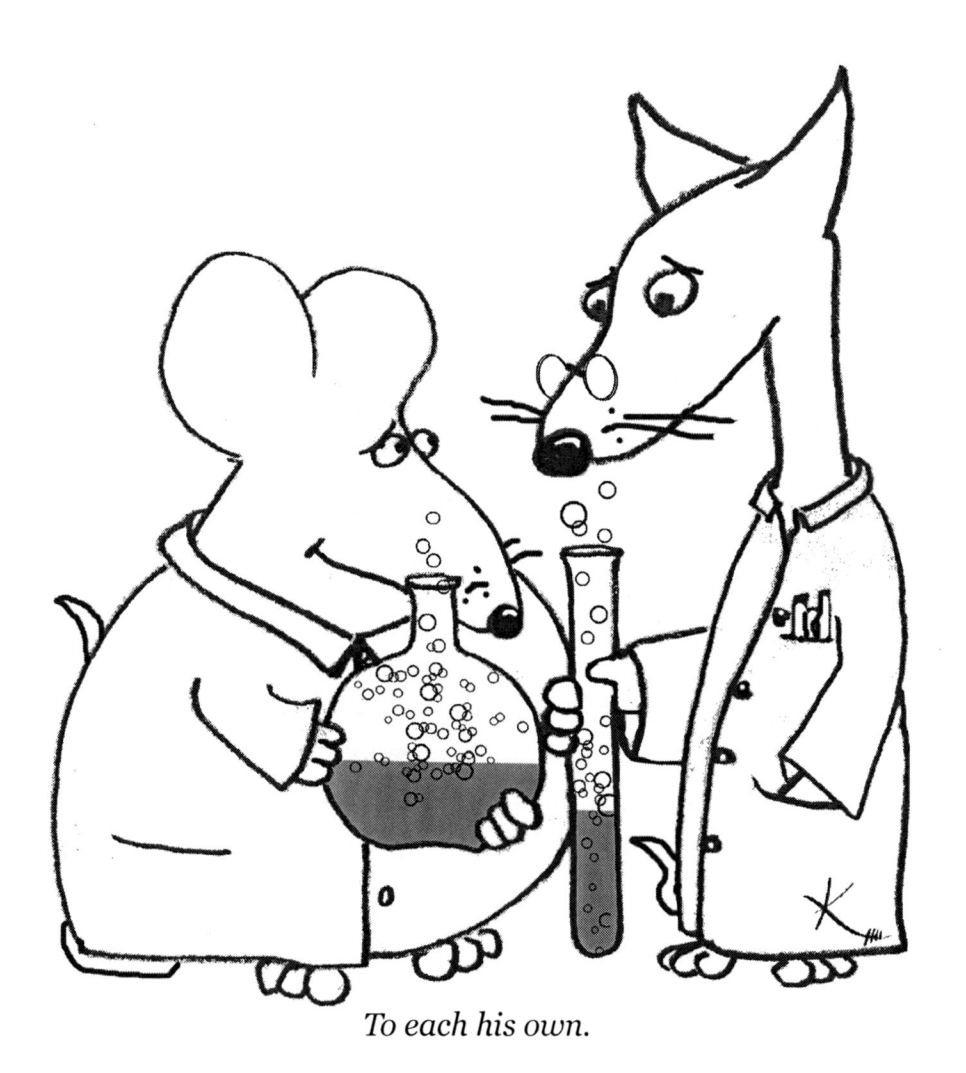

Of Chemicals and Calories

Energy maintenance, like breathing, relies on a series of complex operations that your autonomic nervous system quietly handles for you. To keep you breathing, your brain uses feedback from several receptors to calculate the ratio of carbon dioxide versus oxygen in your lungs before initiating another breath. If this were a conscious effort, could you do the math fast enough to survive?

Similarly, most of the chores concerned with digestion are automatic. When your brain is informed of the smell of freshly baked bread, it immediately sends a signal to your salivary glands. Nerve signals have been clocked at over 500 feet per second so before you know it, you're drooling.

As you sink your teeth into a slab of hot, buttered bread, blood cells rush to your gut like a pack of hyenas descending on a kill. As you chew, you break up the food into smaller particles and mix it with saliva. Saliva acts as a lubricant but it also contains an enzyme called amylase that starts to tear down the chemical bonds that hold starches together.

As the food reaches your stomach, acids tear apart the proteins as fast as they arrive. Bile, stored in the pancreas and secreted by the liver, begins to separate the fats, increasing their surface area so that enzymes have more elbow-room to work.

From end to end, your intestinal tract has receptors for sugars, carbohydrates, fats and other materials. Together, they provide your brain with an operational overview as material moves through your system. Your brain speeds up the process by instructing glands to secrete enzymes that turn food particles into a liquid slush called chyme.

Your brain also sends signals across a network of nerves that surround and penetrate your intestines ordering muscles to contract and release in a series of wavelike maneuvers that massage the food along.

The conversion of food into energy is constant. Over the course of a few hours, nutrients are removed, transported across the intestinal membrane and delivered into the bloodstream for circulation. Anything indigestible is wrung dry of fluids as it squirms toward the exit.

Much of the energy that your gut produces goes to your brain, the hardest working organ in your body. Some energy will be used to repair or replace damaged cells, but if you eat too much, especially if you eat foods high in sugars and fats, your gut produces excess energy that is turned into fat and stored for a rainy day.

Just as soon as your stomach is empty, hormones start signaling for more food and your brain mobilizes its resources for another round of hunting and gathering. Like an assembly line, it must never come to a stop. Where food is concerned, the brain leave nothing to chance. Many would say that it consistently errs on the side of caution.

By itself, this relentless production of calories is not the cause of excess fat, never mind globesity. But it does make you vulnerable to weight gain when you consume more calories than you burn off and if your food is artificially loaded with sugars and fats.

From this perspective, the problem of weight gain seems to be chemical in origin. Therefore the solution must be chemical. Certainly the smart money seems to think so.

Scientists working for the food industry are experts at stimulating your appetite with chemical food additives. The lessons they learn in the laboratory are passed on to marketing experts who use scientific techniques to manipulate your senses and arouse your hunger. Their only objective is to make you eat more of their products and, by golly, they are succeeding.

Meanwhile, biochemists in pharmaceutical companies are looking for ways to counter the effects of their fast-food colleagues. This is no easy task. Selling food products with added sugars, fats, color dyes, odor enhancers, texturizers and preservatives is relatively cheap and simple compared to selling one new drug.

It can take more than ten years and $1 billion dollars to find and test a new drug. Less than 1 in 10 of these drugs will be approved for sale to the public and then it could take five to ten years to reach peak sales and earn a return on investment.

Given the size of the market and the potential pay-off for finding a safe, effective weight-loss pill, most pharmaceutical firms consider the risks worth taking.

Sanofi-Aventis, unlike any of their competitors, put their money on finding a chemical to block cannabinoid receptors and turn off hunger. In general, the scientific community thought this was a bad idea. At the time, there was no evidence that there was such a molecule.

Sanofi reasoned that if a molecule like anandamide exists to turn on appetite, then there should be at least one molecule that does the opposite. If there wasn't, then they would build one.

In 1994, after a decade of searching, Dr. Rinaldi-Carmona and his team at Sanofi Recherche (as it was called then) announced the discovery of a "selective cannabinoid receptor antagonist." It was *selective* because it binds only to cannabinoid receptors. It was an *antagonist* because it deactivates the receptors and prevents signaling.[3] Against all odds, Acomplia had arrived.

28   ACOMPLIA AND YOUR HUNGRY BRAIN

"Facts are stubborn, but statistics are more pliable."
~ Mark Twain

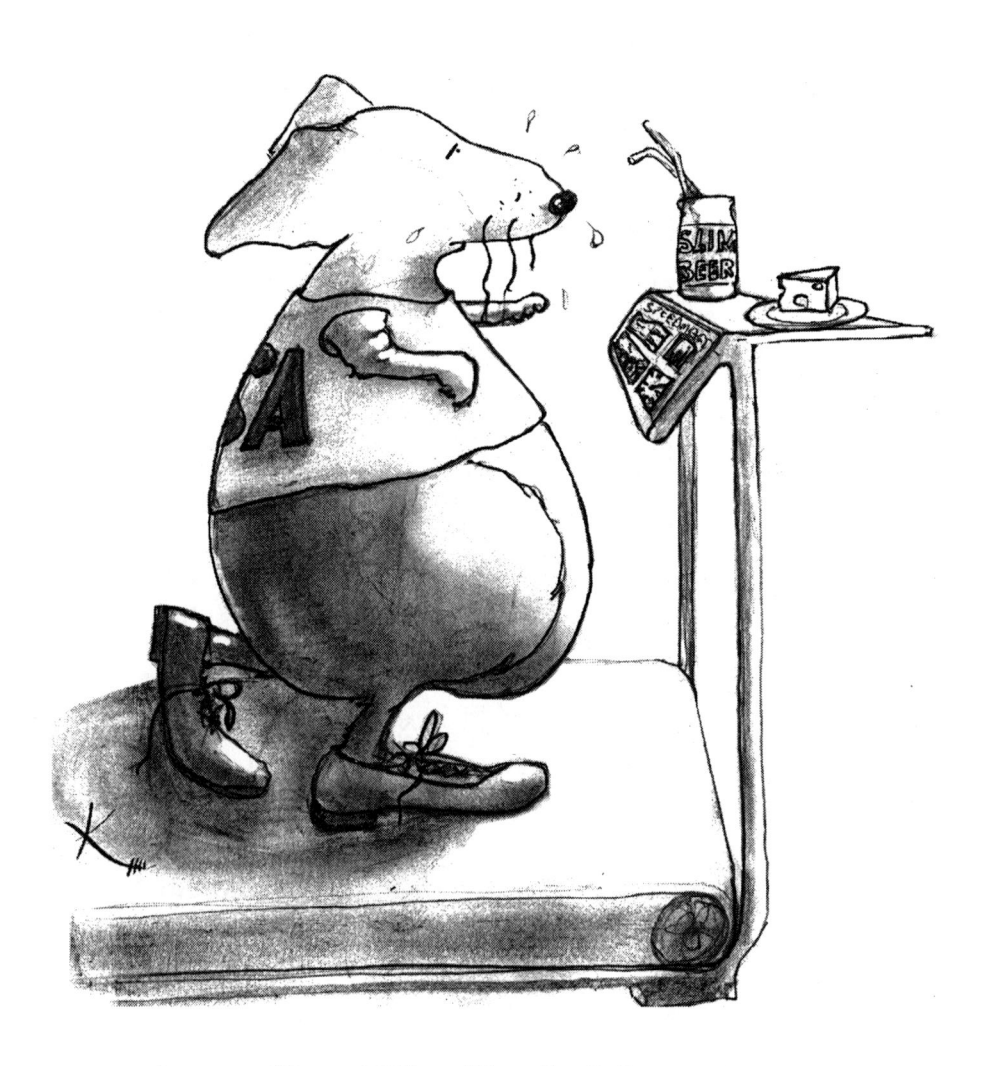

Acomplia – Who Needs It?

America is officially the fattest nation on earth. An estimated 75% are over weight or dangerously obese and as Americans gain weight they increasingly suffer and die from diabetes, heart disease and related cancers. And yet, in the United States, weight gain is not an officially recognized medical condition.

In contrast, the World Health Organization coined the phrase globesity to help sell the notion that weight gain is on a par with such world class diseases as the plague, small pox and HIV-AIDS. The WHO estimates that one billion people around the world suffer from globesity and that the disease is spreading.[4]

To quote Dr. Paul Zimmet, Chairman of the International Congress on Obesity, "the insidious, creeping pandemic of obesity is now engulfing the entire world" and is "as big a threat as global warming and bird flu."[5]

Globesity is a combination of medical circumstances that increases your chances of having a heart attack or developing diabetes. The condition is often referred to as metabolic syndrome because there are physical signs that indicate an underlying disease. The most noticeable sign is excessive body fat, which indicates that something is wrong, but also contributes to the problem.

Not everyone agrees. Some doctors view metabolic syndrome as a collection of separate, identifiable diseases lumped together under one label. Others view it not as a disease, but as a lifestyle choice. None the less, whatever you call it, the symptoms are real and they threaten the well being of people on every continent regardless of age, sex, race or income level.[6,7,8]

Here's why. Weight gain increases your risk of illness due to diabetes, heart disease, stroke, hypertension, gallbladder disease, osteoarthritis (degeneration of cartilage and bone in joints), sleep apnea, breathing problems, breast and uterine cancer and cancer of the colon and the kidneys.[9] Ouch!

The list of disorders does not stop there. If you are over weight you can look forward to a variety of conditions like high blood cholesterol, excess body and facial hair, complications in pregnancy, menstrual irregularities, stress incontinence (urine leakage caused by weak pelvic-floor muscles) and psychological disorders such as depression.

To complicate matters, your doctor could have difficulty diagnosing and treating your illness if you are too heavy. Large patients do not always benefit from x-rays, ultrasounds and MRIs. In the last ten years, the number of useless scans has doubled leading to missed diagnoses and poor treatment.[10]

X-rays, magnetic resonance imaging (MRI) and computer-aided tomography (CAT) results are often discarded because patients are too large. In some cases, like CAT scans, the machine is not big enough to accommodate a patient's extra size. In other cases, imaging fails because rays cannot penetrate deeply enough to be of value. Ultrasound scans are especially unreliable because sound waves cannot always penetrate to the organs.

There are other reasons why you might not receive the best possible care. Over weight patients are more difficult and more costly to treat. Some doctors refuse to take new patients who are too fat because of the extra time and effort involved.

Over weight patients require special facilities and handling, more specialized consultations and assessments plus non-standard treatments and surgeries. Excess body fat increases the risks associated with surgery and can result in further complications.

All of these factors drive up the costs of medical care and your health insurance premiums.[11] In the year 2000, heavier patients are said to have incurred extra medical costs in excess of $117 billion. Many insurance companies now refuse medical coverage to over-weight Americans or charge exorbitant premiums for minimal protection.

Dr. Philip James of the International Obesity Task Force puts it this way: "We are not dealing with a scientific or medical problem. We are dealing with an enormous economic problem that … is going to overwhelm every medical system in the world".[12]

The situation will likely get worse before it gets better because more than 15% of American teens are already over weight.[13] That's triple the number of 20 years ago.

Let's face it, we are getting fatter. Take a moment to measure the distance around your tummy. If you have to unravel more than 3 feet of measuring tape to circumnavigate your waist, you are a candidate for globesity.

Now measure around your hips. If your hips are much bigger around than your waist, that too is supposed to be an indication of globesity.

Another way to assess your risk of globesity is to calculate your Body Mass Index. The BMI is a sliding scale that relates your weight to your height like this:

BMI Formula

$$BMI = \frac{703 \times weight}{height \times height}$$

WHAT'S NEW IN WEIGHT-LOSS DRUGS 33

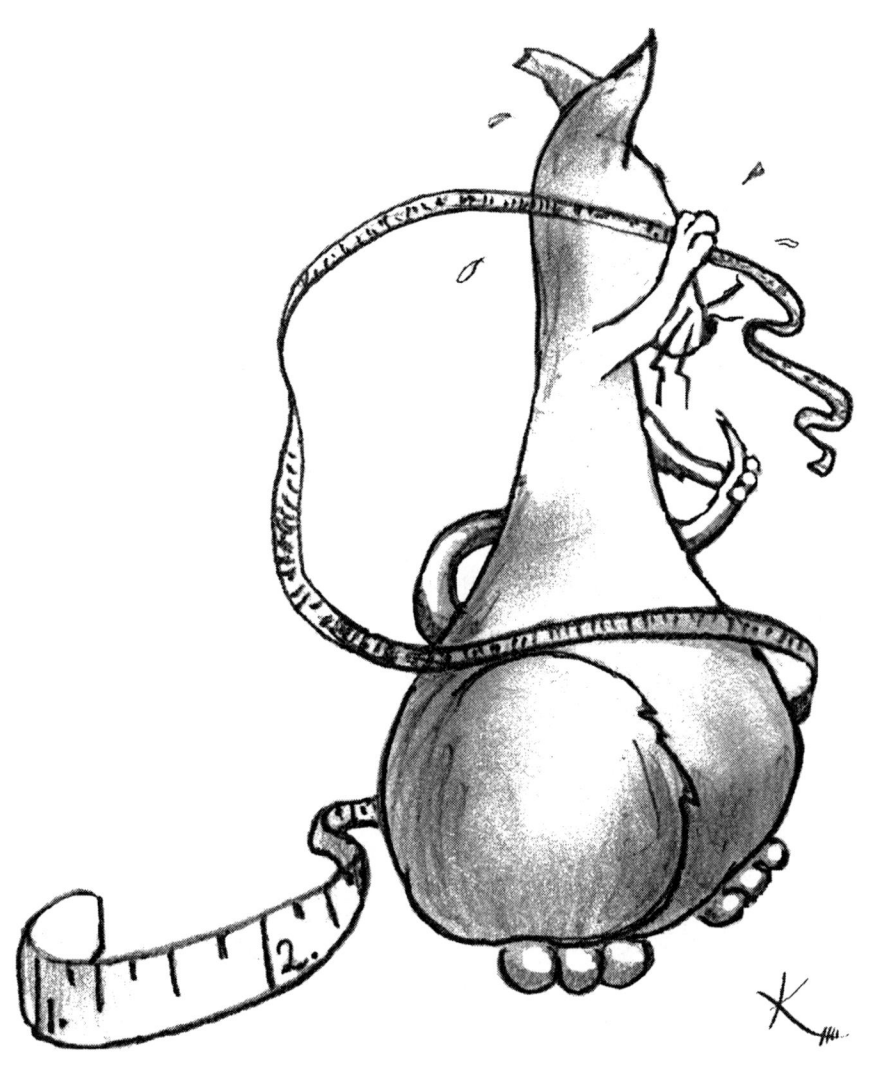

For example, if you weigh 210 pounds and stand 6 feet tall, divide 210 by 72 inches times 72 inches times 703. That works out to 28.5. According to the chart, you are over weight. If your legs get any shorter you'll be obese.

Body Mass Index Chart	
Underweight	under 20
Normal weight	20 to 25
Over weight	25 to 30
Obese	over 30
Morbidly obese	over 40

If your BMI is unflattering, keep in mind that the BMI chart is derived from actuarial tables used by the insurance industry in the 1940's. Those were leaner times.

Take comfort in the knowledge that in 1980 when Arnold Schwarzenegger won his last Mr. Olympia title, he was 6' 2", weighed 260 pounds, and had a BMI of 33.4.[14] By today's standards, he was approaching morbid obesity.

Even if you haven't gained weight in the last fifteen years you might be obese because the National Institute of Health (NIH) revised the standards for the BMI in 1995. Overnight, two thirds of Americans became dangerously over weight and in need of medication.

In the same year, leading experts and prominent doctors, some of them criticized for close ties to the drug and weight loss industry, convinced the NIH to classify obesity as a stand-alone disease requiring treatment.[15] As The Seattle Times put it: "The powerful pharmaceutical industry influences what constitutes a disease, who has it, and how it should be treated."[16]

The NIH was aware that changes to the BMI would inflate the prevalence of obesity, but they claimed to be acting in the public interest because a new generation of weight-conscious consumers would benefit from heightened awareness.[17]

To assess your own risk of globesity you might prefer a more accurate method of diagnosis than the BMI. You might want to ask your doctor to test your fasting glucose, cholesterol and blood pressure levels. After all, blood test results are reliable indicators, aren't they?

WHAT'S NEW IN WEIGHT-LOSS DRUGS 35

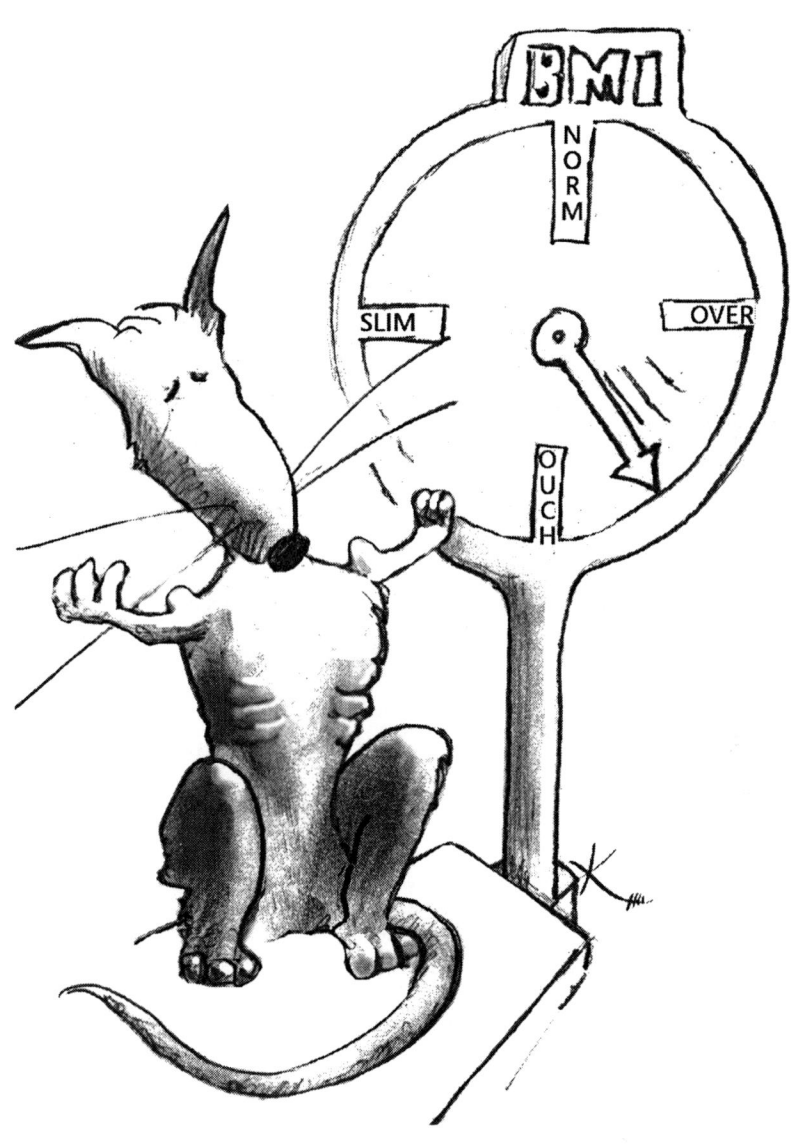

In fact, the disease thresholds of several blood indicators for metabolic syndrome have been lowered by 10% or more. On a morning in 1997, more than 1.7 million Americans would have been shocked to learn that they had become diabetic overnight. Meanwhile, an additional thirteen million people developed hypertension in their sleep.

A year later, due to another adjustment, 42 million people acquired dangerously high cholesterol levels overnight. In all, roughly 75% of Americans were now officially diseased and in need of treatment.

| Re-evaluated Blood Level Indicators ||||
Indicator	Old Level	New Level	Change
Fasting Glucose	140 mg/dL	126 mg/dL	-10 %
Systolic BP	160 mm Hg	140 mm Hg	-14 %
Diastolic BP	100 mm Hg	90 mm Hg	-10 %
Cholesterol	240 mg/dL	200 mg/dL	-10 %

Lowering the blood level indicators was probably a good idea because it helped doctors identify unhealthy trends in time to reverse them. Unfortunately, doctors had only a handful of approved drugs to choose from and all of them had uncomfortable or dangerous side effects.

Pharmaceutical companies were slow to respond to the needs of the market.[18] In the early 1990's, there were only two approved drugs designed to promote fat loss. Fenfluramine, sold under the name Pondimin, was approved in 1973. The other drug, Phentermine, was approved by the Food and Drug Administration (FDA) in 1959, half a century ago.

Fenfluramine increases serotonin levels, a hormone that works on the central nervous system to regulate mood and hunger. Phentermine triggers the release of dopamine and adrenalin, simulating a flight-or-fight response that spurs the rate of metabolism.

A diet-crazed public began combining the two drugs. Doctors, left with no other options, prescribed both drugs together even though the FDA did not approve. Fen-phen, as the combination is called, was a double-barreled appetite suppressant and a very popular weight loss solution.

The off-label use of these drugs presented serious concerns for the FDA. Fenfluramine was increasingly linked to incidents of heart disease and hypertension just as it was catching on as a popular lifestyle drug. Phentermine, an amphetamine, was a stimulant with addictive properties and classified as a controlled substance.

Under public pressure to approve alternative weight loss treatments, the FDA approved dexfenfluramine, a blend of both drugs intended to provide the benefits of Fen-phen without the side effects. Wyeth-Ayerst Laboratories sold it under the brand name Redux, a Latin word meaning resurrection.

Redux was short-lived. In the summer of 1997, doctors at the Mayo Clinic reported 24 cases of abnormal heart valve function among their Redux patients.[19] After alerting doctors and requesting feedback, the FDA received 75 additional reports over the next 2 months. On September 15 of that year, the FDA withdrew both fenfluramine and dexfenfluramine from the market.

Although these patients had no symptoms of heart disease and no obvious distress, Wyeth set up two trust funds for injured consumers as part of a settlement package in expectation of legal claims in excess of $20 billion.

In 1997, the same year that Fen-phen was withdrawn, the FDA approved Sibutramine (Meridia) to control appetite.[20] It offers protection against high cholesterol and diabetes but can lead to dry mouth and sleeplessness.[21] Some patients experience a dangerous increase in blood pressure so the use of Sibutramine remains a calculated risk.

In 1999, the FDA approved another drug called Orlistat, better known by its brand name Xenical. Orlistat reduces fat absorption by roughly 30% by preventing enzymes from breaking down fats during digestion.[22] Orlistat has its own list of side effects: diarrhea, stomach bloat, oily spotting, gas with discharge, fecal urgency, fatty/oily stools and frequent bowel movements.

While these complaints are distressing, they are not life threatening and may actually help you lose weight because the sheer discomfort they cause will definitely change your attitude toward food.

Sibutramine works on the brain, which may account for the scope and severity of its effects. Orlistat, with dramatic but less dire consequences, tackles the other end.

Two other drugs that almost made it to market were Axokine and Topamax. Axokine is an example of a drug with early potential that had to be scrubbed during human trials. Topamax, prescribed originally for epilepsy, promotes weight loss but was abandoned due to issues involving the central nervous system.

Synthetic leptin was once promising as a treatment for weight gain. Natural leptin is a hormone that curbs appetite and gets its name from the Greek word *leptos*, which means thin. In 1994, experiments with leptin and over weight mice lead to the discovery of the ob gene, short for obesity gene, which provides the genetic information needed to make leptin.

Mice with a mutated version of the ob gene were unable to make leptin so they ate too much and became obese. When mice with normal ob genes were given extra leptin they ate less and lost weight, suggesting that raising leptin levels would be a good treatment for obesity in humans. The idea being that if a little leptin is good, more should be better.

Initially, reports were hopeful. In 1997, researchers at Tufts University reported that volunteers lost four times as much weight on leptin as those on a placebo.[23] The higher the dose, the greater the weight loss. Sadly, no one else has been able to duplicate their results and leptin has fallen out of favor.

Despite the drawbacks associated with current weight-control drugs, sales in the U.S. still exceed $550 million per year. Pharmaceutical companies are anxious to expand their market, but since the withdrawal of Fen-phen and the crippling financial damages suffered by Wyeth, they were forced to explore new approaches.

In February of 2007, Alli (pronounced ally) was the first drug ever to win approval as an over-the-counter treatment for weight gain.[24] Why? Was this a revolutionary new drug? No, it was simply a low dose version of Orlistat that one consumer advocacy group called "a dangerous mistake".[25]

Meanwhile, it is easier to sell products that stimulate appetite rather than control it. Chemists in the food industry invent new and enticing foods on a regular basis. They frequently enhance the flavor and texture of these products with sugars and fats that are known to alter your blood chemistry, clog or damage your arteries and physically alter your brain cells.

When rats eat too much sugar they get excessive amounts of fatty acids in their blood and livers in just four weeks.[26] After 20 weeks, they are grossly over weight and fatty acids have spread throughout their bodies, collecting in both muscle and fat tissue. These are the same fatty acids that cause diabetes in humans.

It's fair to say that you are not meant to ingest large quantities of sugar any more than rats are. And yet, prepared and packaged foods are loaded with it. From alcohol to zabaglione: sugar sells.

We could subject sugar to the same rigorous testing as medical drugs. We could insist on proof that it does no harm. But if we go down that road, where do we stop? One day, you might need a doctor's prescription for pretzels and beer!

An alternative solution would be a safe, effective drug that protects you against symptoms of globesity, reduces your food intake and provides immunity from constant cravings.

Hundreds of new drugs are in development to fill that need, but Acomplia is among the first to be approved for human use. It represents an innovative approach to weight loss that is winning supporters in Europe and elsewhere, but remains controversial and unavailable in America.

WHAT'S NEW IN WEIGHT-LOSS DRUGS

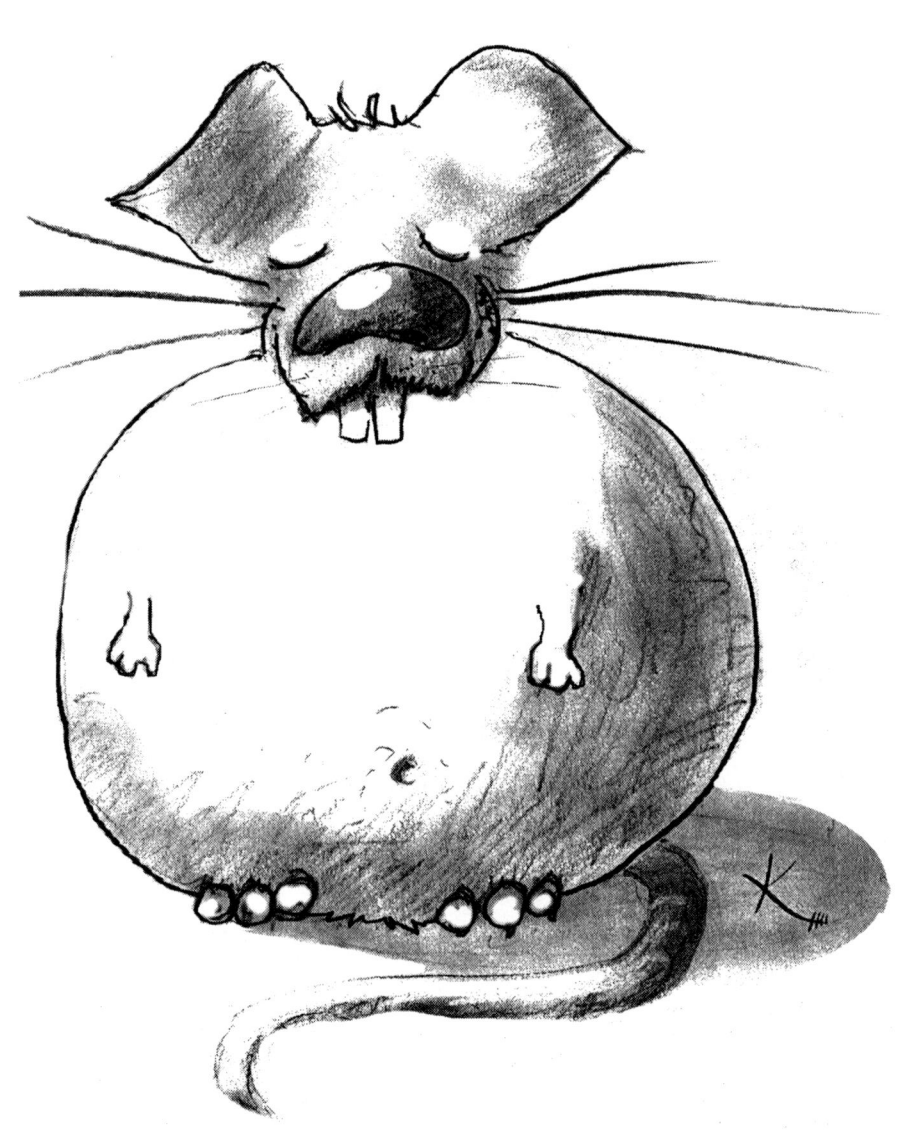

Ob Mouse

*"The trouble with resisting temptation is that
it may never come your way again."*
~ Korman's Law

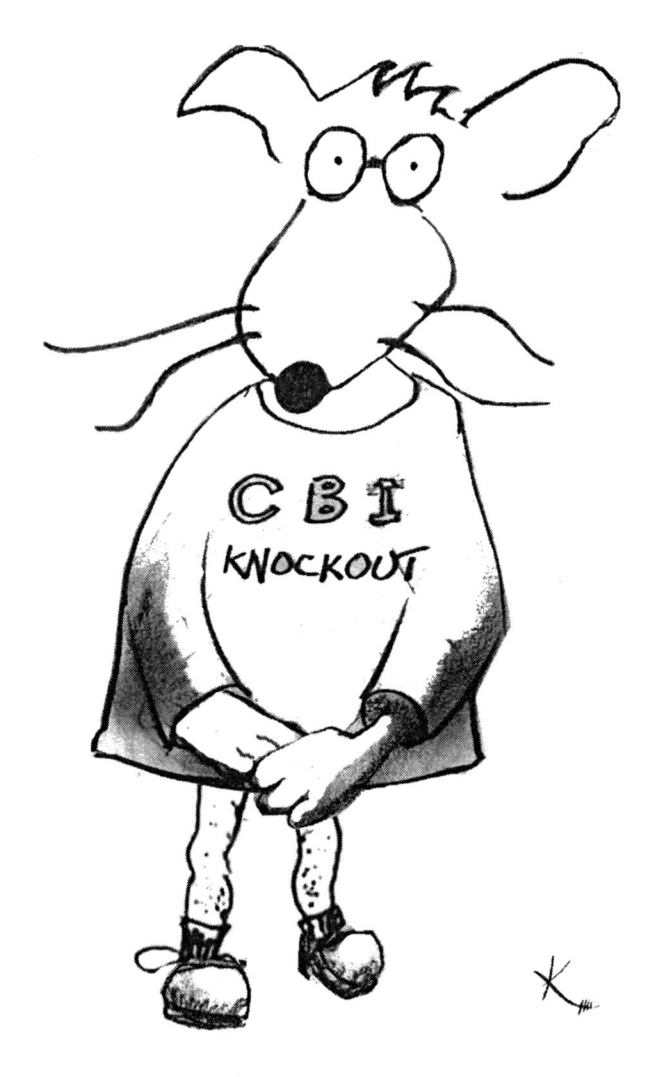

Missing Genes

Acomplia - Does It Work?

Acomplia does one thing very well: it locks onto type 1 cannabinoid receptors and turns them off. That is all Acomplia really does. It's what happens next that makes all the difference.

Type 1 cannabinoid receptors (CB1 receptors) grow on many brain cells, including those of your midbrain. This location is important because the midbrain is a cross-roads of neural traffic concerned with thirst, hunger and pleasure as well as more primitive responses like fear, aggression and sexual arousal.

Your CB1 receptors talk to your brain constantly, providing a steady stream of information that is necessary to manage your body's energy needs. Acomplia interrupts that conversation.

In early animal experiments, treatment with Acomplia led to a number of surprising results. Food moved more quickly through the digestive tract. Blood contained fewer fatty acids. The metabolism sped up. Excess energy was burned off as heat. The body produced additional adiponectin, a hormone that fights fat.

These results were very encouraging, but such a wide range of effects was confusing. Was Acomplia selective and binding to CB1 receptors alone or was it interacting with a number of different receptors?

Acomplia had to prove that it was not promiscuous because drug makers need highly selective molecules that are dedicated to a single receptor. A drug that binds to multiple receptors can have multiple effects that are more difficult to understand and predict, let alone control.

The best way to test Acomplia is to see what happens when it is introduced into an animal with no CB1 receptors. If nothing happens, then Acomplia is selective. If changes do occur, then Acomplia probably does bind to other receptors. All this experiment needs is an animal careless enough to misplace its CB1 receptors.

WHAT'S NEW IN WEIGHT-LOSS DRUGS   45

Enter the CB1 knockout mouse. He doesn't wear boxing gloves or fancy silk shorts and to look at him you would not guess that he is a product of genetic engineering, a mutant conceived in a test tube.

In all ways, the knockout mouse is like any other mouse except for one thing – he doesn't own a pair of genes. The very genes he needs to make CB1 receptors were "knocked out" using a method known as gene splicing.

Genes come in pairs, one from dad and one from mom. They contain assembly instructions that determine the number and location of all your receptors. Today, biochemists can use enzymes to snip open the DNA at just the right spot to remove the recipe for CB1 receptors.

There are many enzymes available for gene splicing because biochemists collect enzymes the way squirrels gather nuts. They even have an enzyme, called a ligase, that knits the snipped ends of DNA strands back together again.

This experiment, like all good experiments, required a control group in order to provide a basis for comparison. For that reason, wildtype mice were chosen to participate in parallel to knockout mice.

A wildtype is the same as a knockout mouse except that it was conceived by natural means and has all its genetic bits and pieces intact. In spite of the name, wildtype mice are born in captivity where they enjoy subsidized housing and regular meals.

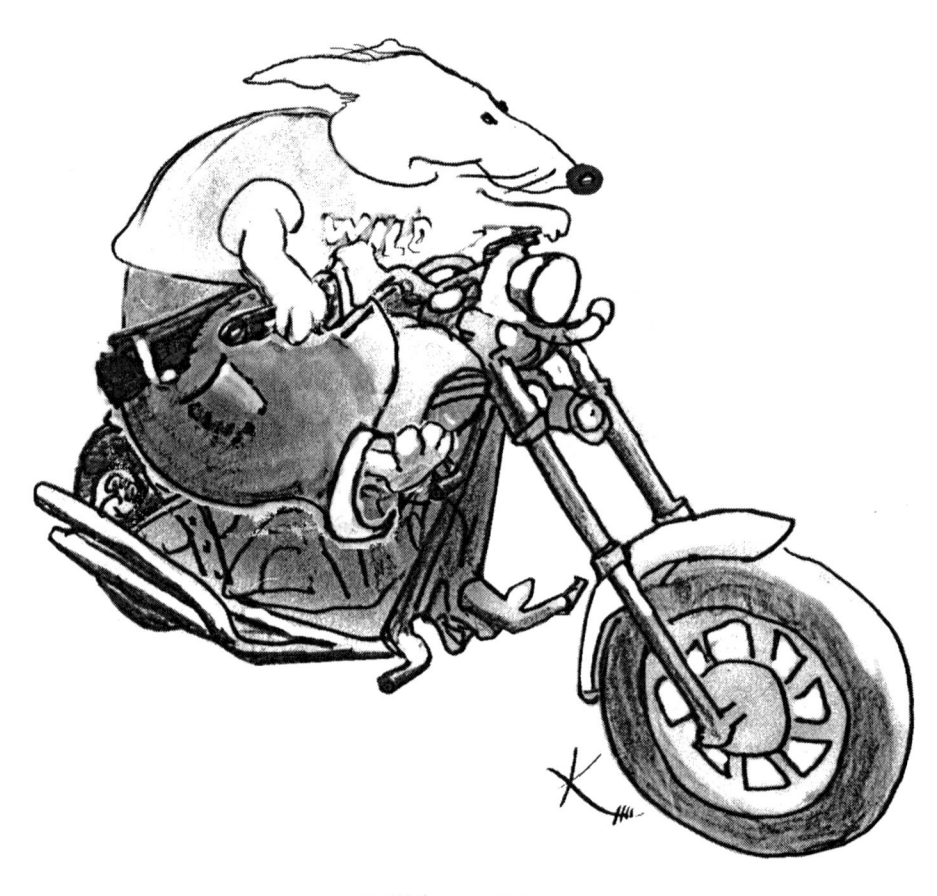

Wildtype Mouse

To set up the experiment, knockouts and wildtype mice were subjected to a period of food rationing. As food became scarce, wildtype mice desperately ate all the food they could get their little paws on. In contrast, knockout mice were content to nibble and displayed no change in their feeding behavior at all.[27]

When treated with Acomplia, the wildtype suddenly remembered their manners and appeared less frantic and less hungry but knockout mice displayed no change in their feeding behavior one way or the other.

That appears to settle the question. Acomplia has no effect whatsoever when CB1 receptors are absent. Therefore, Acomplia is selective - it binds only to CB1 receptors.

The problem here is that scientists rarely find evidence for something if they are not looking for it. Acomplia did not alter the appetites of knockout mice, but how do we know it did not affect their mood or cause a loss of memory? There could be side effects that no one has thought to investigate.

One important thing we do know from this experiment is that the cannabinoid system tends to promote hunger all by itself. That's not too surprising because the cannabinoid system is a survival mechanism common to all mammals.

Did you notice, however, that removing all the CB1 receptors only reduced the appetite of hungry mice? It did not eliminate it. It looks very much as if the cannabinoid system is not alone in stimulating hunger.

Many biological processes have back-up systems that prevent a total shut-down of essential services. This is probably the case here. But you have to wonder - if Acomplia fails to overcome hunger for regular lab chow, how will it ever control cravings for really tasty treats loaded with sugar?

That's a good question. The answer may surprise you. First of all, CB1 knockout mice do not care for sugar.[28] They can take it or leave it. If you remove CB1 receptors you may as well take away the sugar. Researchers actually have trouble training knockout mice to eat sweet food instead of regular chow. That's like having a child who prefers turnips to ice cream! Is it possible that the desire for sugar depends on an active cannabinoid system? Let's find out.

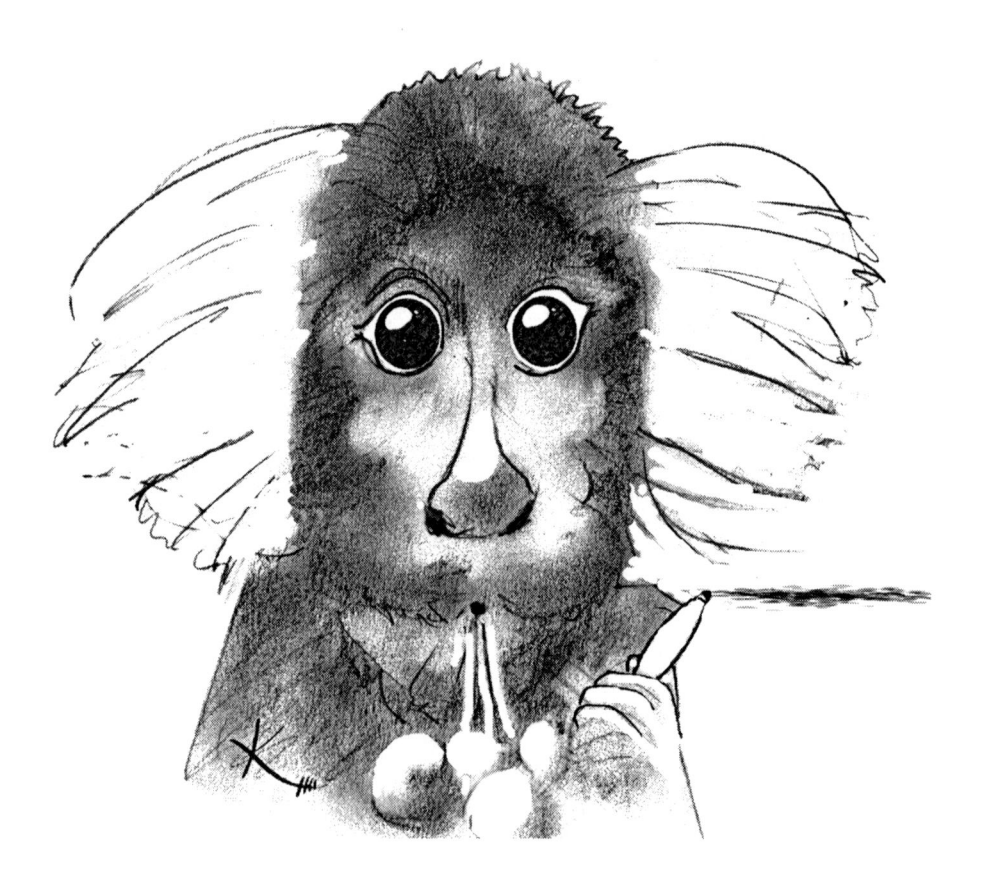

Marmosets are cute, little monkeys with bright eyes and a sweet tooth. When they get high on marijuana they get very excited at feeding time and eat more than usual. Nothing turns them on more than their favorite treat. A combination of THC and cane sugar sends them into a feeding frenzy.[29]

After a dose of Acomplia, they completely change their behavior. They lose interest in food, eat less often and less intensely and refuse extra offerings of cane sugar. Higher doses of Acomplia reduces their food intake by another 30%.

Again, Acomplia did not eliminate hunger, but it was effective against THC and sugar combined. Acomplia has the same effect on other animals including hungry rats, fat rats and skinny rats, stoned or otherwise.[30] Without doubt, Acomplia does reduce appetite and food intake even when the food is sweet and highly appealing.

Okay. Cutting back on portions and avoiding calorie rich foods with the help of Acomplia might prevent weight gain, but what about weight loss. Appetite control is one thing, but can Acomplia actually reverse weight gain and remove body fat.

I thought you'd never ask. Here's what happened to some extremely fat mice weighing in at a whopping 0.9 pounds, about 46% more than normal. They had high blood levels of leptin, insulin and glucose - all the symptoms of metabolic syndrome.[31]

A third of them were free to eat as much rich, tasty food as they wanted. Another third were restricted to a meager portion of standard chow. The last third had open access to the same rich food that made them fat in the first place, but they also took a daily dose of Acomplia.

Over a period of ten weeks, the first group steadily gained weight. The rationed group, as you would expect, lost 26% of their body weight. But here's the good news: the last group lost 24% of their body weight in spite of their poor diet. Taking Acomplia produced the same results as strict rationing.

But wait, there's more. After 10 weeks on Acomplia, the mice experienced renewed health. Leptin levels were down by 81%, insulin by 78% and glucose by 67%. Triglyceride levels also dropped and cholesterol ratios improved.

In brief, Acomplia reversed weight gain in mice who ate excessive amounts of fats and sugars; it reduced symptoms of metabolic syndrome; and it restored obese mice to reasonably good health.[32]

These were exciting results, but they were puzzling because Acomplia had a much stronger effect than anyone expected. Neither a drop in food intake nor an increase in physical activity adequately explained the total weight loss experienced by Acomplia mice.

We now know that Acomplia initiated a ripple effect that flowed downstream to other systems that also contributed to weight loss. Here a some examples.

Active cannabinoids do more than cause hunger, they slow down food as it travels through your gut so that it is digested more completely and produces more calories.[33] By aiding digestion, cannabinoids increase energy input and promote weight gain.

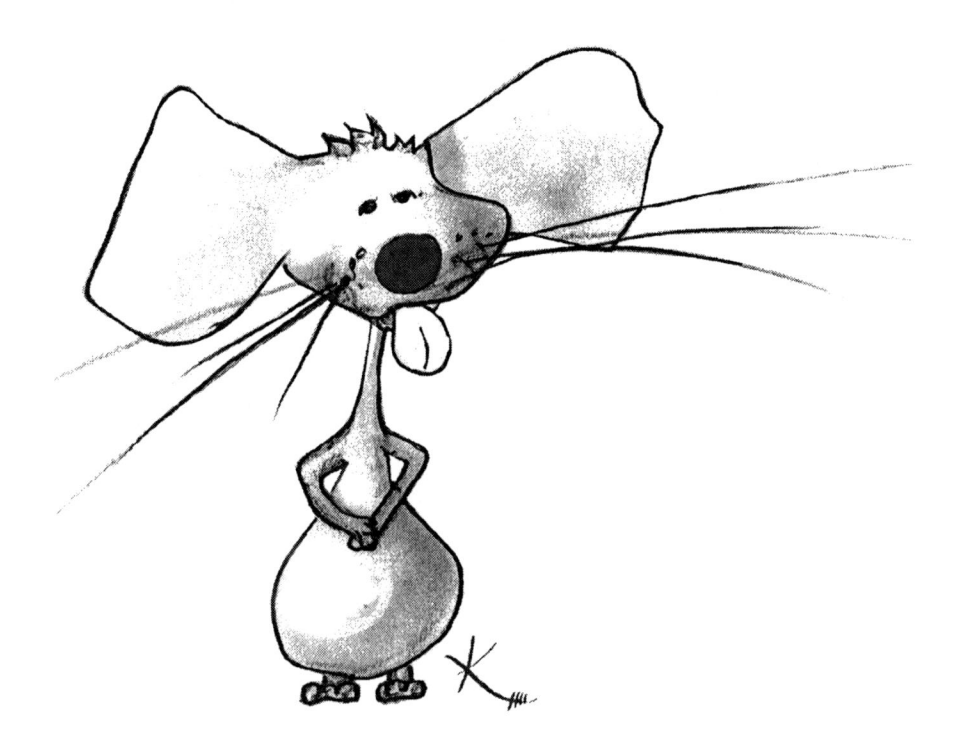

Acomplia has the opposite effect. It speeds up motility from 60% to 75% by accelerating peristalsis, the muscular action that squeezes food through your intestines, and reduces calories.

But there's a catch. Chubby mice become tolerant to Acomplia after 8 days (3 days in some cases) and the effect wears off. Tolerance occurs when receptors stop responding unless they receive ever-increasing stimulation. One of nature's little jokes is the tendency of marijuana to induce both hunger and constipation at the same time.

Our natural tolerance for THC prevents matters from coming to a sticky end. But if mice tolerate Acomplia, then some people may too and they won't experience Acomplia's full benefits.

Another way that Acomplia reduces weight gain is entirely different. This may sound a bit far fetched, by it looks as though Acomplia can burn off excess energy reserves.

The soleus is a powerful muscle that runs from the heel to the back of the knee. It keeps us from falling flat on our faces when we stand up.[34] In rats, it is a very active muscle that uses up more than its share of oxygen and glucose. Yet, after seven days of treatment with Acomplia, it consumes 37% more oxygen than usual and increased its glucose uptake by an additional 68%.[35]

That is remarkable. These are the kind of changes in metabolism normally associated with exercise. Either Acomplia burns energy or these rats secretly enrolled in ballet class!

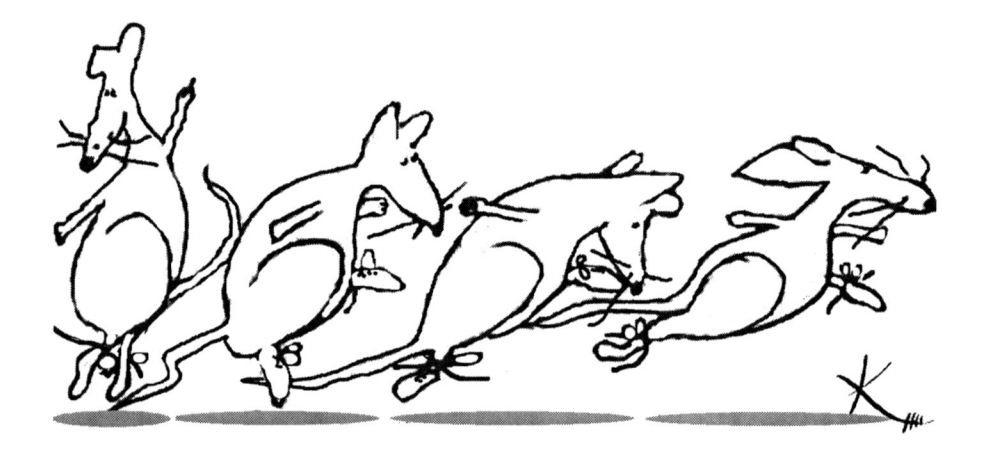

While taking Acomplia, these rats ate less, lost weight and kept the weight off for five days after treatment. The research team concluded that "Acomplia has a direct effect on energy expenditure" that increases metabolic rate and burns off excess energy in the form of heat, what biologists call thermogenesis.[36]

Another way Acomplia promotes weight loss is by increasing the availability of adiponectin.[37] You might not be familiar with this hormone. The name comes from the Greek word *adiponecrosis* which means fat-death. Adiponectin literally breaks down stored fats.

In humans, low levels of adiponectin are linked to metabolic syndrome, in part because diabetics have lower adiponectin levels than non-diabetics. Odd as it seems, fat cells are the source of adiponectin, the agent of their own demise. Stranger still, the fatter you get, the less adiponectin you make. A similar problem with leptin suggests that these two hormones work together to keep thin people thin and fat people fat.

Their is hope that this conspiracy can be foiled. Bathing fat cells in Acomplia forces them to manufacture extra adiponectin, which in turn should reduce body weight, restore insulin sensitivity and lower glucose levels.

Acomplia, as you can see, promotes weight loss in unexpected ways. There are bound to be more surprises in store because CB1 receptors have been discovered in your other brain, not the one in your head, but the smaller one you keep in your gut.

Your enteric nervous system (ENS) is a network of a billion neurons that monitors and controls your entire gastrointestinal system. At this point we can only guess what the implications of this discovery will be.

As for your big brain, in the next chapter we explore how Acomplia reduces cravings and alters eating habits by literally changing your mind.

Part Two

The Usual Suspects

"There is no sincerer love than the love of food."
~ George Bernard Shaw

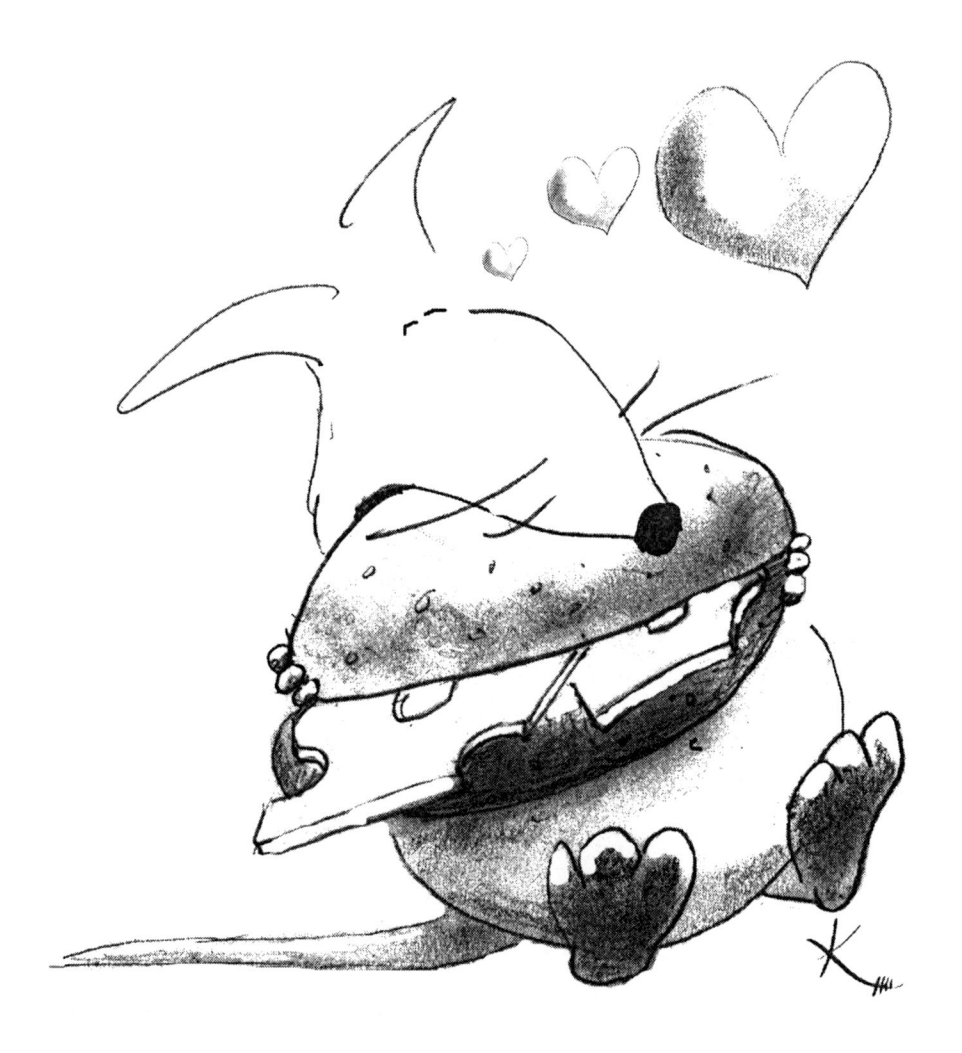

Dopamine - Signals of Desire

Having children can be an exhausting, inconvenient and dangerous business. And that's just conception! Mating is an essential biological activity, but as Lord Chesterton once said, "The pleasure is momentary, the position ridiculous, and the expense damnable."

Sex requires a high degree of motivation otherwise organisms would rather not expend the energy. The same could be said of feeding. No matter how fleeting, fattening or financially draining, the pleasure food brings is irresistible.

Food, or just the promise of it, triggers the release of hormones and neurotransmitters that offer incentives and rewards that ensure you remember to eat regularly. One of the most persuasive of these is a neurohormone called dopamine.

Your desire for sex or food depends on dopamine. People with low dopamine levels tell us that they like the taste of food but have no appetite for it. They also admit that they still enjoy sex but have no special urge for it. They feel no compelling need to either breed or feed.

If you have chronically low dopamine levels you could experience a lack of gusto in your life. To compensate, you might try binging, gambling and risk-taking, compulsive behaviors that stimulate dopamine release. Some people turn to substances like nicotine, heroin and marijuana for the same reason.

Most of us associate dopamine with pleasure, but experts are fairly certain that dopamine is not the actual cause of good feelings, but rather an essential ingredient that sets the stage for pleasant sensations.

Happy rats have high levels of dopamine in the midbrain. Take away dopamine and they become lethargic and incurious. Yes, they eat less and lose weight, but they also lose their playfulness and generally seem depressed.

Acomplia blocks signals that contribute to dopamine release and reduces dopamine activity in the brains of rats.[38-39] If this leads to depression, the rats aren't talking, but we'll look into this in more detail further on.

For now, just be aware that dopamine affects your desires, your motivations, your physical movement and your sense of joy and excitement. It makes it possible for you to learn and to remember all those things that are important to you.

Dopamine makes it possible for different parts of your brain to collaborate. It helps your emotional midbrain influence your rational forebrain. For instance, if you decide to stop breathing for a while or refuse to take food and water, your midbrain will nag like a back-seat driver until you give up these dangerous ideas.

Sometimes, these communications aren't so helpful. You could sensibly decide to quit smoking, but your addicted mind won't like that idea either. It will apply physical and emotional pressure to dominate your logical mind at the merest hint of cigarette smoke. If you smoke, you are hyper-sensitive to nicotine clues and, thanks to dopamine, your midbrain recognizes the smallest details linked to gratification.

The point is, dopamine is critical to the creation of memories and the ability to recall them. It helps record incoming sensory data and store the information for future reference. If the information leads to a reward, additional dopamine is secreted to reinforce the memory.

Bigger rewards release more dopamine and form stronger memories. As you repeatedly access the same rewarding memories, your brain cells grow new dopamine receptors to strengthen the connection, making you a more efficient pleasure seeker.

Obviously, dopamine secretion is far too important to be controlled by cannabinoids alone. Important processes usually have a back-up and in this case your opioid system is more than equal to the task.

Rats and humans share several natural opioids, like enkephalin, which normally regulates pain, but can be used to make rats eat up to six times more food than usual.[40]

Rats and humans also respond to opioids added to our food. Both enjoy the taste of sugar and tend to eat more sweet food than is good for us because sugar excites opioid receptors, increases dopamine production and provides a sense of pleasure.

But there is a problem with sugar and its effect on the opioid system. If you take sugar away from rats who are accustomed to it, they get anxious. Their teeth chatter and they get the shakes just like human addicts suffering withdrawal.[41]

The implication is that sweetened foods flood your system with dopamine and lead to addiction. In other words, signals of desire precipitate a cascade of chemicals that wash over your brain and trigger a call to action that we recognize as cravings.

*"Strength is the capacity to break a chocolate bar
into four pieces with your bare hands –
and then eat just one of the pieces."*
~ Judith Viorst

WHAT'S NEW IN WEIGHT-LOSS DRUGS 63

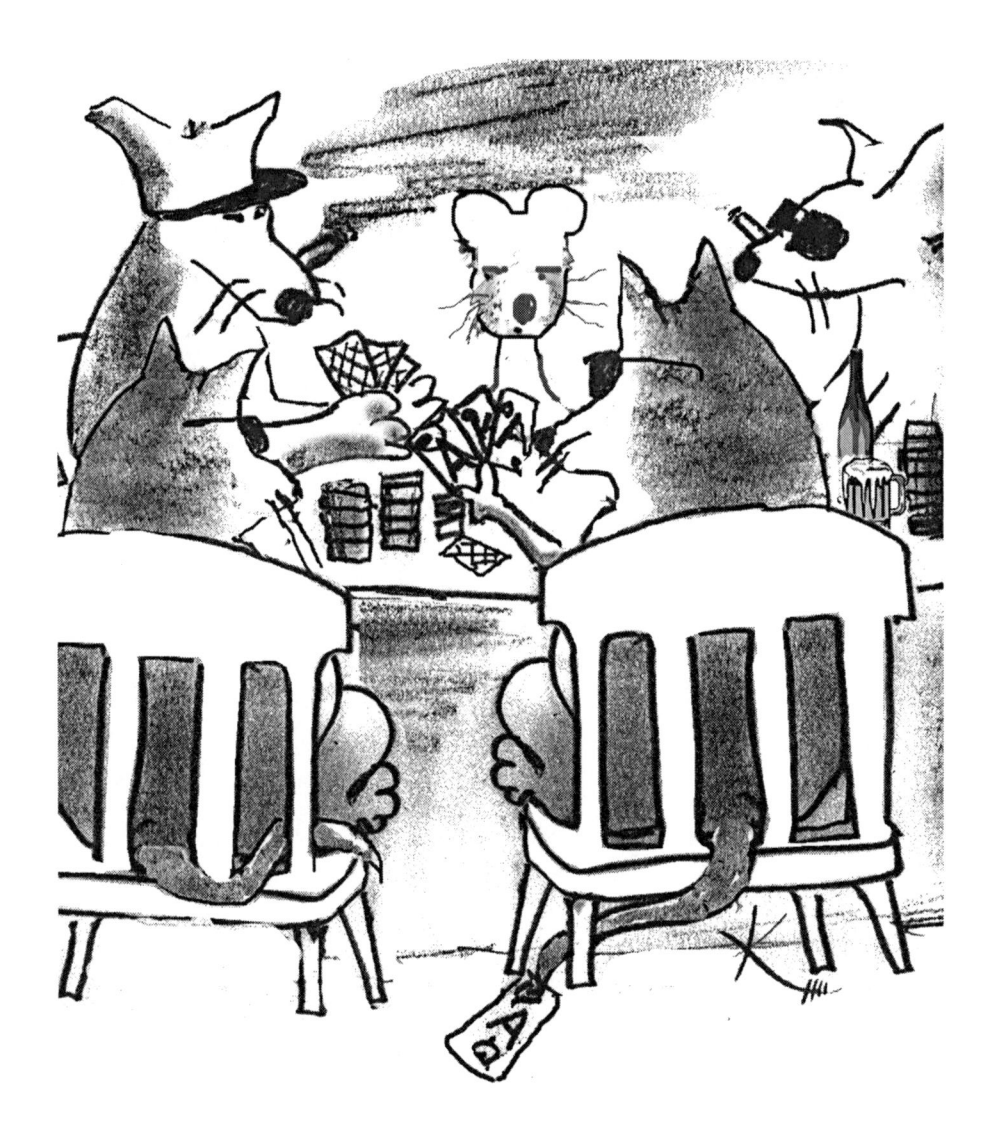

Cannabinoids – Old Dog, New Tricks

Your brain has trained your body to do tricks for food. It uses the same method you would use to teach your dog to roll over or fetch. It rewards you with pleasure if you behave; it punishes you with hunger if you do not.

Thanks to media hype, you could have the impression that Acomplia is a miracle drug and that all you have to do is pop a tiny pill and before you can say 'N-piperino-5-(4-chlorophenyl)-1-(2,4-dichlorophenyl)-4-methylpyrazole-3-carboxamide' all those nasty cravings go away. Is it really that simple?

After taking Acomplia, rodents with a habit of compulsive feeding reduced their food intake and slimmed down. Some animals, usually excited by sugar, became indifferent to it. Rats addicted to nicotine stop seeking it and others addicted to alcohol went on the wagon.

Acomplia achieved these results by turning off CB1 receptors in spite of an array of natural cannabinoids whose job is to turn them on. Anandamide, the bliss molecule, is the best understood. Another is 2AG (short for 2-arachidonyl-glycerol). There are several more whose names are almost as long as this sentence.

Cannabinoids are instruments of survival. They are necessary to so many biological processes that they are found in mammals, birds, fish and reptiles. Your entire metabolism is completely dependent on cannabinoids. They may be few in number, but they are indispensable.

As you know, cannabinoids regulate dopamine production through your CB1 receptors. This is an extremely important function because it affects your ability to learn and to remember. You could say that cannabinoids influence who you are and what you think.

Because CB1 receptors grow abundantly all over your brain, cannabinoids affect signaling in the amygdala, the center of fear and aggression; the hippocampus where memories are formed; and the prefrontal cortex where your plans and thoughts take shape.[42]

Cannabinoids also operate in areas of motor control and help regulate blood pressure and heart rate as well as thirst, hunger and sexual arousal. They report directly to the hypothalamus, a central knot of nerves that manages your body's energy needs.

They aid communications between different parts of your brain, integrating billions of neurons into a synchronized network capable of sustaining life and consciousness.

In 2001, researchers were startled to discover how powerful cannabinoids could really be. When they washed brain cells in anandamide, it caused an immediate drop in the production of adenylate cyclase.[43] This is significant because adenylate cyclase helps produce the chemicals your nerves require for signaling.[44] By cutting off the supply of adenylate cyclase, anandamide directly impeded the signaling capacity of other systems.

What's more, adenylate cyclase is a critical component of learning and memory, which implies that cannabinoids have a firm grip on the central nervous system to the point that they can manipulate what you learn and how well you remember it.

In part, this is due to the strange effect cannabinoids have on your brain cells when they engage your CB1 receptors. After binding to anandamide, CB1 receptors duck beneath the surface of the cell's membrane where no other molecules can reach them.[45]

For some reason, once a few of them disappeared, the other receptors on the cell's surface go into hiding.[46] In effect, a few cannabinoid molecules can hijack every receptor in the vicinity without having to bind to each and every one of them.

Tactics like these, suppressing competitive signaling and monopolizing CB1 receptors, demonstrate the power of cannabinoids. Now take into account that they operate within those brain structures responsible for emotion, behavior and long term memory and you begin to understand how hunger and cravings can be so overwhelming.

For all these reasons, cannabinoids are very good at teaching you to sing for your supper. How, then, does Acomplia overcome the strangle-hold that cannabinoids have on CB1 receptors?

Firstly, one of the reasons that cannabinoids are so effective is due to the nature of CB1 receptors themselves. CB1 receptors are coupled to G-proteins, which makes them very efficient.

G-protein coupled receptors are usually involved whenever you get sick. Lucky for you, because over half the drugs sold today target this type of receptor. G-protein coupled receptors stick out above the surface of a cell so they are easier to find. They are also small enough to bind to simple, man-made molecules used in medications.

Acomplia, a relatively simple molecule, not only fits into CB1 receptors, it aggressively digs out cannabinoids and takes their place. Once embedded, it takes advantage of the receptors abilities to rapidly restore signaling and adenylate cyclase levels.

Then it forces all hidden CB1 receptors back to the surface where it can get at them.[47-48]

How Acomplia does this is a mystery, but one thing is certain: Acomplia does not merely obstruct cannabinoids, it dominates them. Does that mean Acomplia can turn off your cravings? Sorry, it really isn't that simple.

*"If you're not having fun,
you're doing something wrong."
~ Groucho Marx*

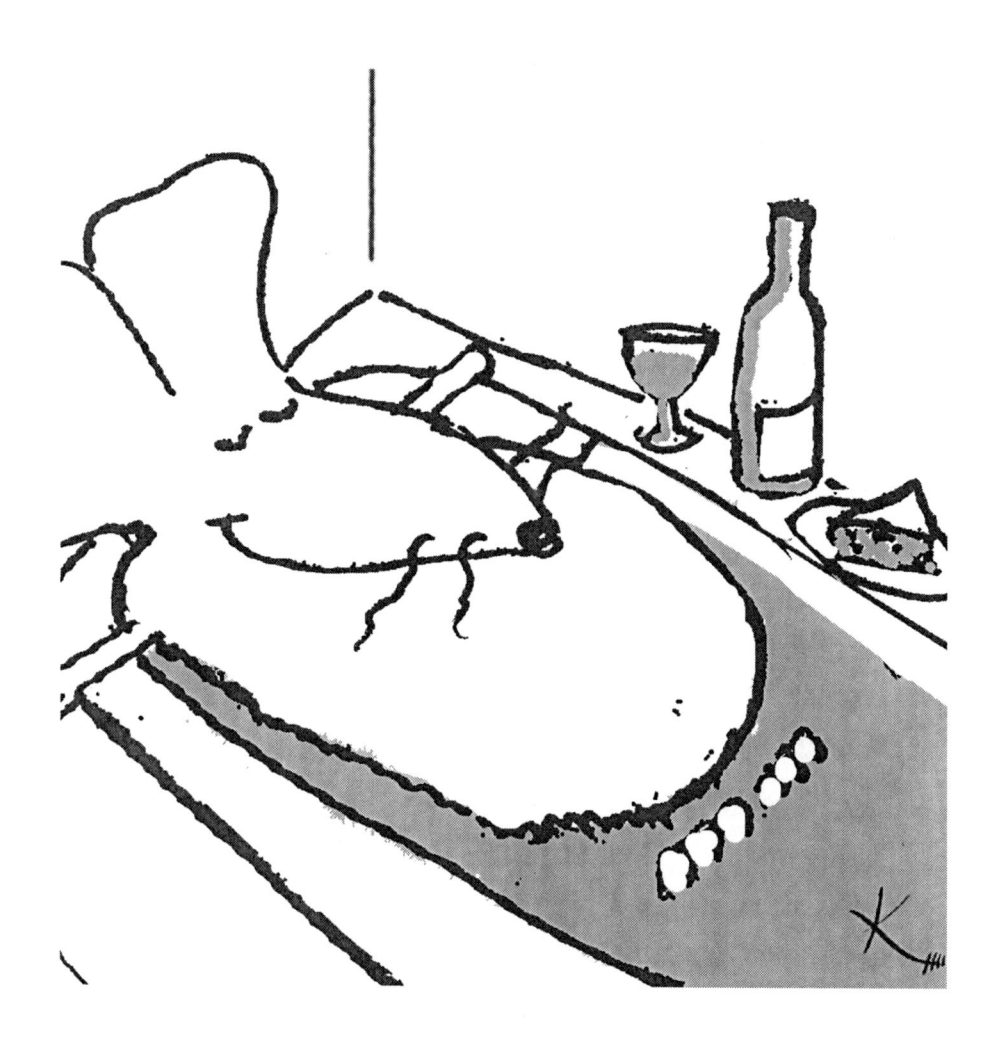

Opioids – Resistance is Futile

Once upon a time, there were some rats who spent their lives in comfort and relaxation.[49] They enjoyed the benefits of regular room service, clean bedding and fresh water, all in a climatically controlled environment. They exercised regularly and they ate sensibly. They were, by any measure, healthy and satisfied.

One day, some of these rats received a drop of anandamide, the bliss molecule, just under the skin. They abruptly forgot their table manners and crowded around the dinner table demanding second helpings. Larger doses of anandamide eventually turned them into insatiable gluttons and in the following weeks they rapidly gained weight.

To counter this, they were given Acomplia. That didn't accomplish much although higher and higher doses did produce a corresponding drop in food intake. The fact remained, anandamide was driving them to eat too much.

In another experiment, the rats usually they ate dinner just before lights out and had no interest in food once they were tucked in for the night.[50] After taking THC just before bed time, they shuffled about in the dark in their little rat pajamas searching for midnight snacks.

As in the previous experiment, Acomplia reduced overeating, but anandamide and THC continued to stimulate hunger. Since the CB1 receptors were turned off, they must be acting through some other type of receptor. But which kind?

We know that anandamide puts mice into a trance and prevents them from responding to mild electric shock or warming themselves when temperatures drop. It does this by activating opioid receptors to regulate pain sensitivity and motor control.[51]

We also know that opioid receptors bind to morphine, from opium plants, to reduce appetite. Morphine is used medically for pain relief, but not as a weight-loss treatment because it is very addictive and causes disturbing side effects like lethargy, drowsiness and nightmares.

WHAT'S NEW IN WEIGHT-LOSS DRUGS

So opioid receptors look like the obvious culprit. Let's do those two experiments again, only this time, we'll use a drug called naloxone that sticks to opioid receptors like tar on a road.

Naloxone literally scrubs molecules out of opioid receptors and prevents them from coming back. It can completely displace heroin or morphine from a drug addict's brain in under two minutes. In previous experiments, naloxone was nearly twice as effective as Acomplia at reducing hunger caused by THC.[52]

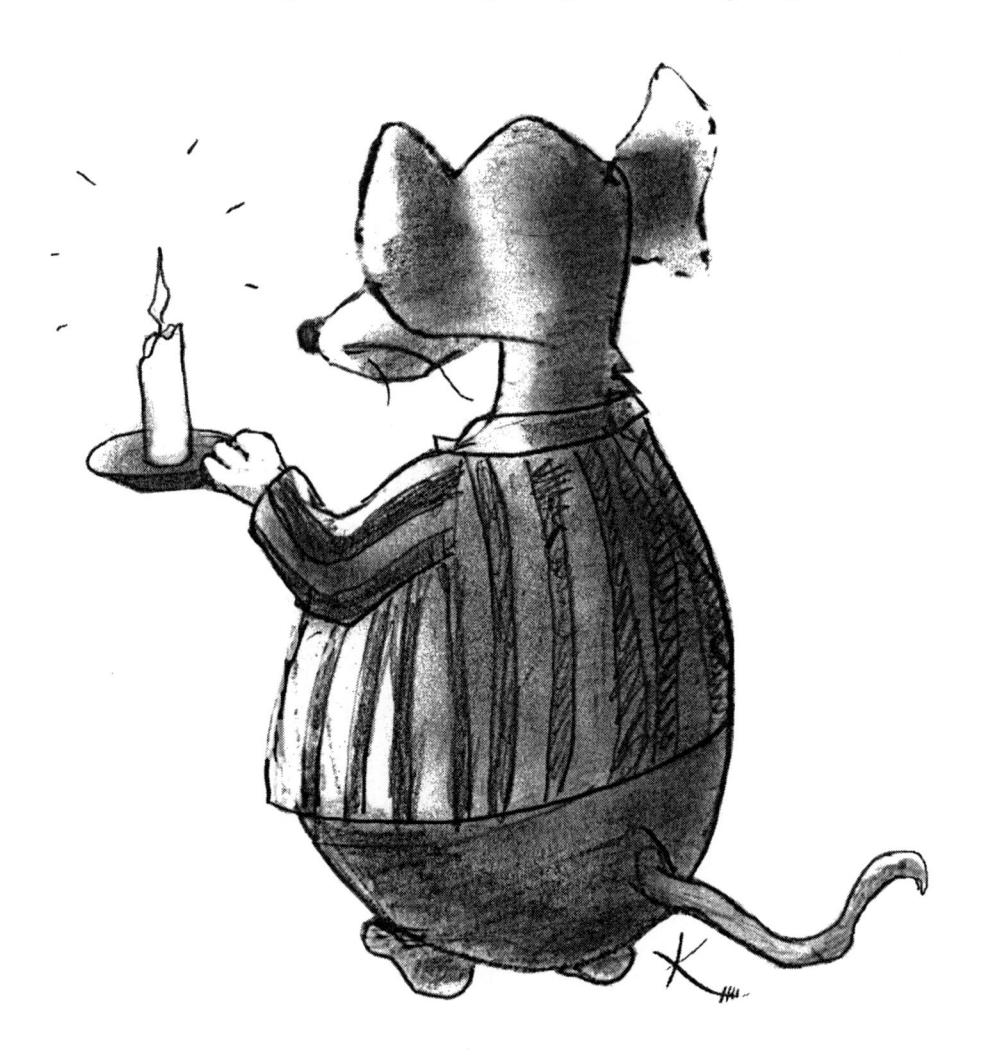

Repeating the experiments with naloxone and Acomplia together reduced food intake by 73%, a combined effect greater than either drug could achieve alone against either THC or anandamide.

This tells us that cannabinoid and opioid receptors are in cahoots. Either one of them can trigger our need to feed. Turning them on makes well-fed rats hungry.[53] Turning them off makes even starving rats lose interest in food.[54] Because they work together, it takes the super-additive effective of two drugs to dramatically reverse feeding.[55]

There are some important side notes to these experiments. First, Acomplia was effective when taken orally. Second, its effects were relatively long lasting, up to three days in some cases. Third, Acomplia did not interfere with water intake.

These are important consideration when marketing any new drug because consumers like you would probably prefer to swallow a single, long-lasting pill than a get a needle and an enema every 24 hours.

Knowing that the cannabinoid and opioid systems are integrated and that they collaborate to motivate and reward feeding, you can understand why dieting can be so difficult and why will power seems almost irrelevant.

WHAT'S NEW IN WEIGHT-LOSS DRUGS 73

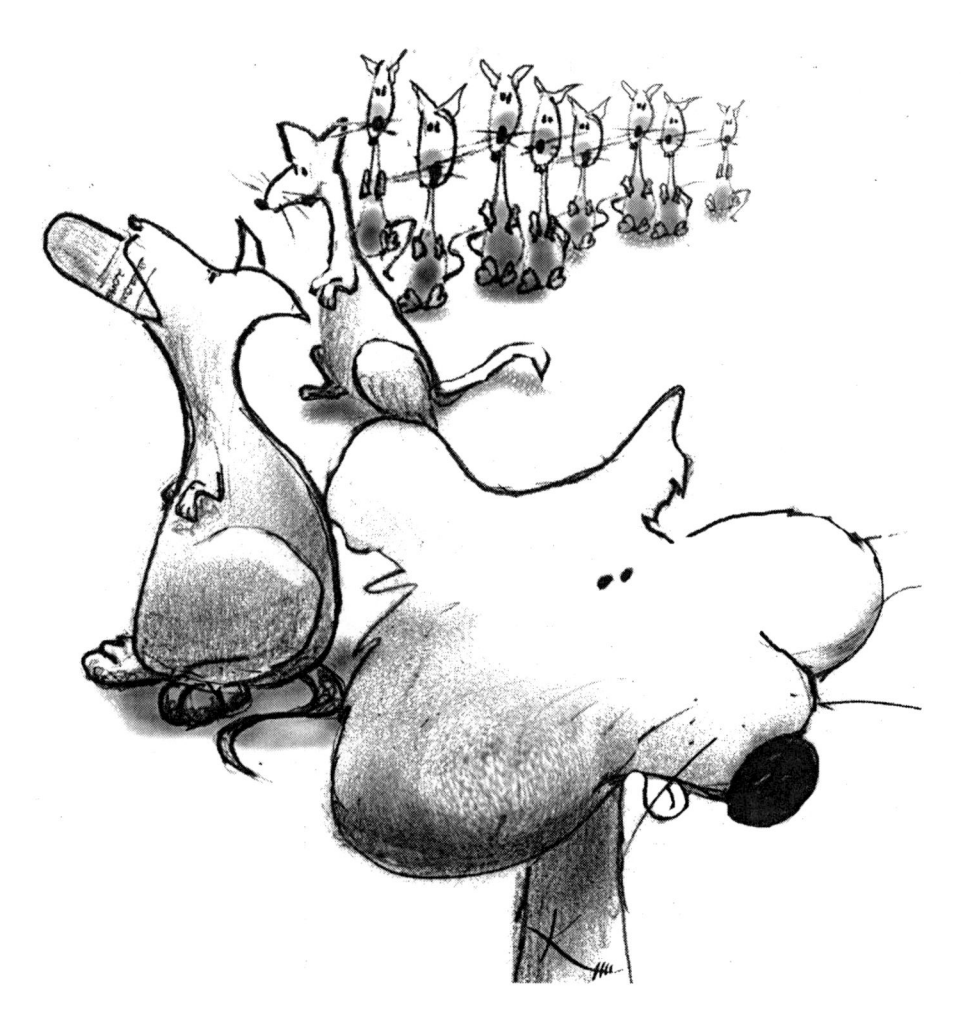

Oral Medication Reduces Food Intake

"The only way to keep your health is to eat what you don't want,
drink what you don't like,
and do what you'd rather not."
~ Mark Twain

WHAT'S NEW IN WEIGHT-LOSS DRUGS

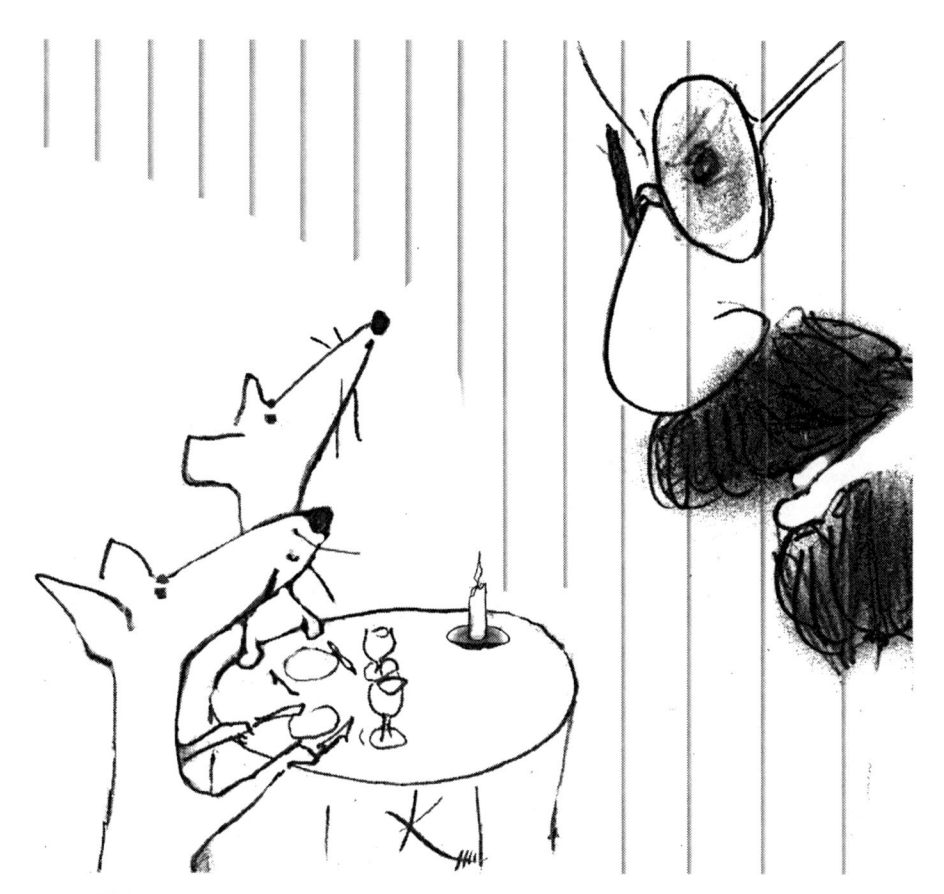

We'll have the Mozzarella Bufala with the '98 Chianti Riserva

Cravings – Addiction Lite

In the early days of clinical psychology, cravings were considered to be *an impairment of the will; an emotional state* or *an abnormal impulse* that is *a characteristic factor in mania*. Today, cravings are no longer a sign of mental disorder, but the basis of a sound economy.

Packaged and processed foods earn more than $3 trillion annually.[56] As the U.S. population surpasses 300 million, we now have 5% of the world's mouths to feed, yet our grocery bill exceeds 30% of global spending.[57]

Why do we spend so much on food? Many nutritionists and doctors claim that prepared foods contain excessive amounts of sugars and fats that are naturally addictive. Sugars and fats overstimulate our cannabinoid and opioid systems and cause cravings that can nag incessantly or strike with the intensity of sexual desire.

That could be why many of us make unhealthy food choices, even when we know better. Here is an experiment that demonstrates the difference between satisfying your energy requirements and satisfying your need to eat.

If you put a rat into a box with little windows cut into one wall, he will poke his nose through the openings out of sheer curiosity. If he is consistently rewarded with a pellet of food for looking out one of the windows, he quickly catches on.

If the rules change and require two nose pokes in the correct window to earn one pellet of food, then four nose pokes, then six and so on, the rat will adapt. Some rats have learned to optimize their earnings at an average rate of 100 pellets per half hour.

Rats can do the math, so when the food service deteriorates to the point that the reward is simply not worth the effort, they give up trying. This is called *the break point*.

In one experiment, rats went on strike after 166 nose pokes earned a mere 10 pellets. What would it take to push them beyond this point?

That's right, over-stimulate their cannabinoid and opioid receptors with a little THC. The effect is so stimulating that rats push well past their usual break point. It takes a combined dose of Acomplia and naloxone together to bring the break point down again.

In people it's the same. Your cannabinoid and opioid systems overlap and your desire to eat is greatest when both types of receptors are over-stimulated. Magnetic resonance imaging (MRI) of the human brain during food cravings reveals that most of the action occurs in three main areas and that the pattern of activity is identical to that of drug addiction.[58]

One hot spot is the caudate, a hub of signaling activity that lights up an MRI screen when you are in love.[59] You have two caudates, one in each hemisphere, which are active whenever you get emotional or expect a reward.[60] They are involved with memory, learning and motor control. You rely on them to help you locate the ice cream, figure out how to open the packaging and manipulate your spoon.[61]

Another area is the insula cortex, which lights up when addicts are exposed to environmental clues that trigger cravings for drugs, alcohol or nicotine. Smokers who suffer a stroke that damages their insular cortex are often cured of their addiction to cigarettes.[62]

The third is the hippocampus, an old part of the brain that creates new memories, particularly spatial memories necessary for navigating.[63] This is one of the first areas to falter in people who suffer from Alzheimer's disease. In animals and humans it is essential for locating food sources.

All three areas are important to learning, memory, mobility, emotions and the search for food. They are physically and chemically connected by nerve fibers to each other and to the decision making regions of your brain. Millions of nerve cells provide connective tissue and encourage cross-communications. When active, they light up the brain like a Christmas tree.

Another part of the brain that gets excited by food is the nucleus accumbens. This is often called the pleasure center of the brain and gets its Latin name from the way it leans like a drunk against a lamp post.

The accumbens releases dopamine as a reward for eating. It also rewards sex. It even rewards you for playing video games. When stimulated by electrodes, the nucleus accumbens provides so much pleasure that rats obsessively press an activation lever until they die of exhaustion.[64]

Oddly, Acomplia appears to have no effect on the nucleus accumbens.[65] That's a concern because food loaded with sugars and fats tends to excite the nucleus accumbens and intensify cravings. Sugars and fats change your brain and alter your behavior in subtle ways. Are they turning you into a wired rat who eats, not for survival, but for gratification?

WHAT'S NEW IN WEIGHT-LOSS DRUGS

A growing number of doctors believe that metabolic syndrome and globesity are just fancy names for food addiction. As with other addictions, willpower alone is not likely to change your habits. Addiction is not about character – it's about chemistry.

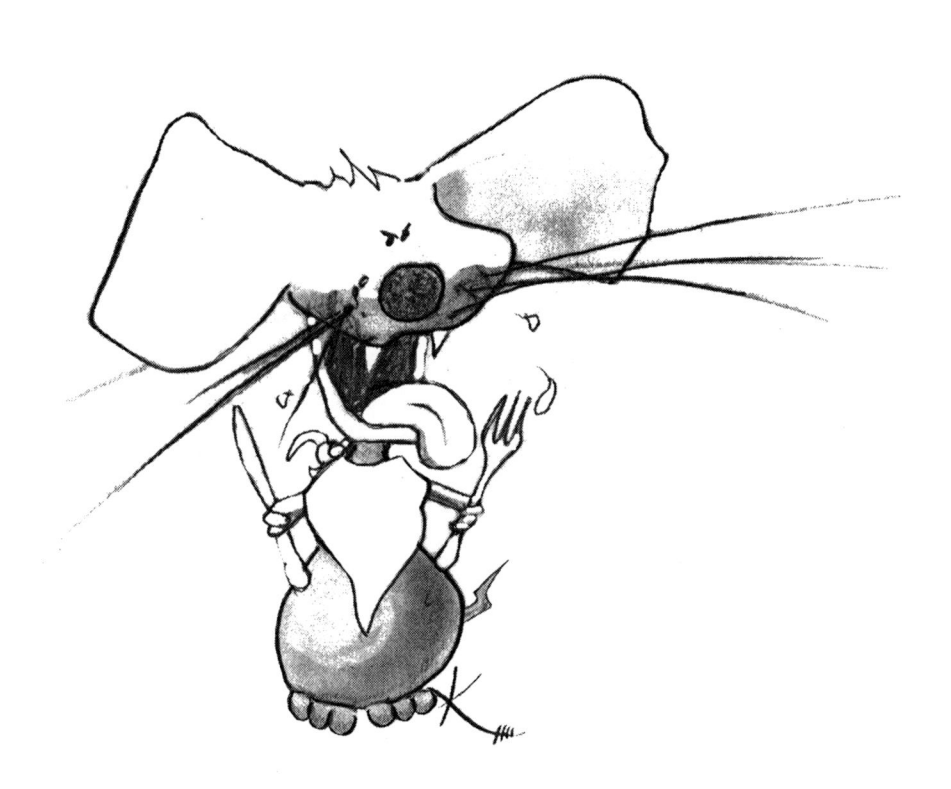

"A full belly makes a dull brain."
~ Benjamin Franklin

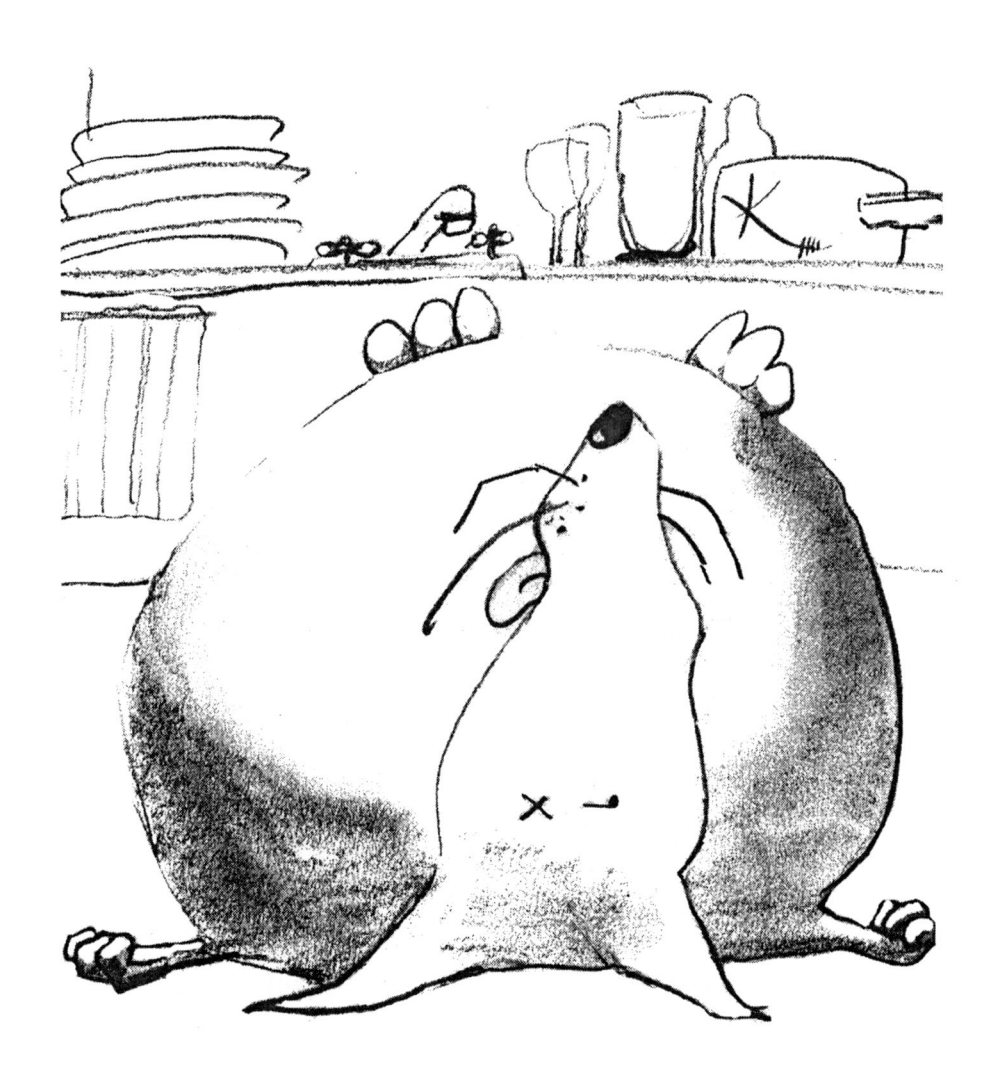

Melanocortins – Your Secret Ally

Did you ever polish off a big meal and feel so sleepy afterwards that you could barely keep your eyes open? Did you feel as if your brain had turned to mush and your legs to jelly?

Chances are you experienced postprandial hypotension. You might want to practice saying that a couple of times - it's a great excuse to avoid doing dishes. Even a slight drop in blood pressure after a meal can leave you feeling dizzy and faint. This is no time to be handling sharp objects and fragile dinnerware!

Blame it on your cannabinoids. They are strong vasodilators, which means they can turn stiff blood vessels into limp spaghetti.[66] An overly active cannabinoid system contributes to hypotension (low blood pressure) and possibly hemorrhagic shock (loss of blood to the brain or vital organs).[67]

If your blood flow slows down too much, your brain and heart may starve for oxygen and you will pass out. Without emergency services you could go into shock and have a heart attack.

Your immune system will respond to the emergency by producing monocytes (white blood cells) and platelets (blood-clotting agents), but the same process also produces more cannabinoids, which only makes matters worse.

A few years ago, some rats experienced such an extreme drop in blood pressure that they went into shock and had only minutes to live.[68] Once anandamide was identified as the culprit, treatment with Acomplia restored their vital signs to normal resulting in a 100% survival rate.

A follow up study of rats with lethally low blood pressure confirmed that Acomplia increases arterial pressure, pulse pressure and respiratory rate - three critical factors in the prevention of shock.[69]

Tests show that Acomplia can raise the heart rate sufficiently to avoid a sudden drop in blood pressure.[70] Furthermore, it protects epithelial cells from damage, keeping blood vessels strong and healthy. And combining Acomplia with an opioid blocker reverses hemorrhagic shock more effectively than either one alone.[71]

These are wonderful benefits, but they are also untidy. Unexpected results, even good ones, mean that a drug is not well understood. Why is Acomplia having an effect on blood pressure? The most reasonable explanation is that a third system has become involved.

The most likely candidate is the melanocortin (MC) system, which produces hormones involved in some of the most important functions in your body. MC hormones help determine your sexuality, your growth rate and your ability to socialize and find a mate. They also affect your memory.

Despite the importance of the work they do, MC hormones are small and fragile and are usually referred to as MC peptides. Peptide being a Greek word for *digestible*, correctly suggests that they are rapidly broken down, especially in the digestive tract.

That said, MC peptides are still capable of carrying signals through the blood stream. It's possible they act as go-betweens, shuttling messages to and from the opioid and cannabinoid systems and other parts of the brain. That would help to explain why the MC system appears to operate in parallel.

The MC system is extremely complex and, as far as we know, has at least five types of receptors. A malfunction of the MC4 receptor is of special interest because it is the most common form of genetic mutation found in over-weight children. A child with this mutated gene may not be a binge eater or look obese until later in life. As less than 3% of children have this mutation, it is certainly not the cause of globesity.[72]

Still, experiments with mice reveal that MC4 receptors definitely influence feeding and weight gain. MC4 knockout mice are inactive, eat too much and become obese.[73] If the missing receptors are restored using gene therapy, the obesity rate drops by 60%.

On the other side of the coin, rats with active MC4 receptors eat less than usual. A dose of Acomplia causes them to eat less again.[74] All by itself, the MC system reduces feeding, but it has a much stronger effect in combination with Acomplia.

The best explanation for this is that Acomplia prevents excessive cannabinoid signaling, allowing the MC system to operate more actively. This could explain why Acomplia sometimes has a positive effect on hypotension.

In the future, there may be a pill you can take after dinner to avoid a sudden drop in blood pressure. Until then, if you are not ready to take your turn at the kitchen sink, repeat this phrase: postprandial hypotension. It works like a charm.

WHAT'S NEW IN WEIGHT-LOSS DRUGS 85

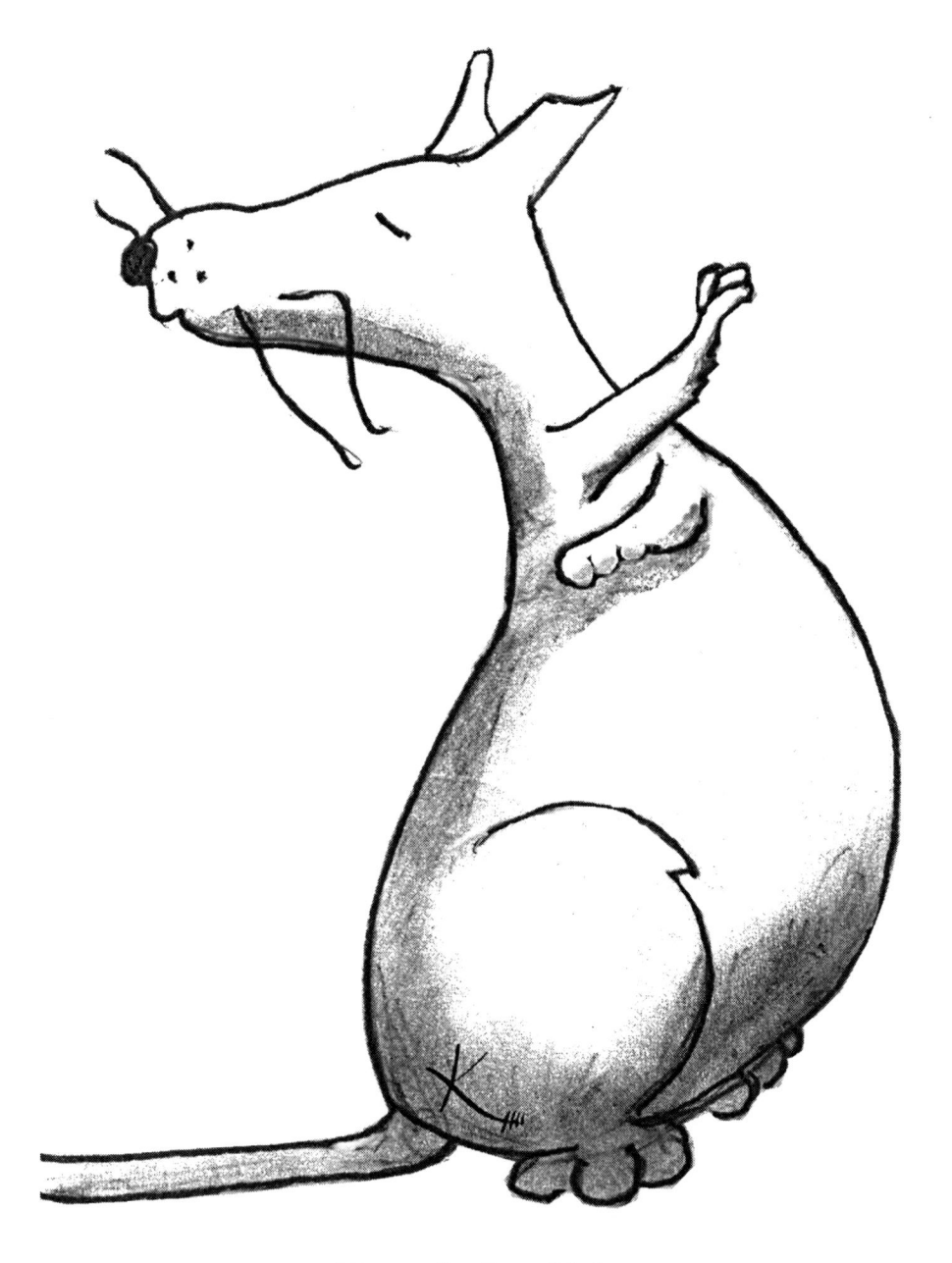

No, really, I couldn't.

PART THREE

THE TRIALS OF ACOMPLIA

*"All my life, I always wanted to be somebody.
Now I see that I should have been more specific."
~ Jane Wagner*

WHAT'S NEW IN WEIGHT-LOSS DRUGS   89

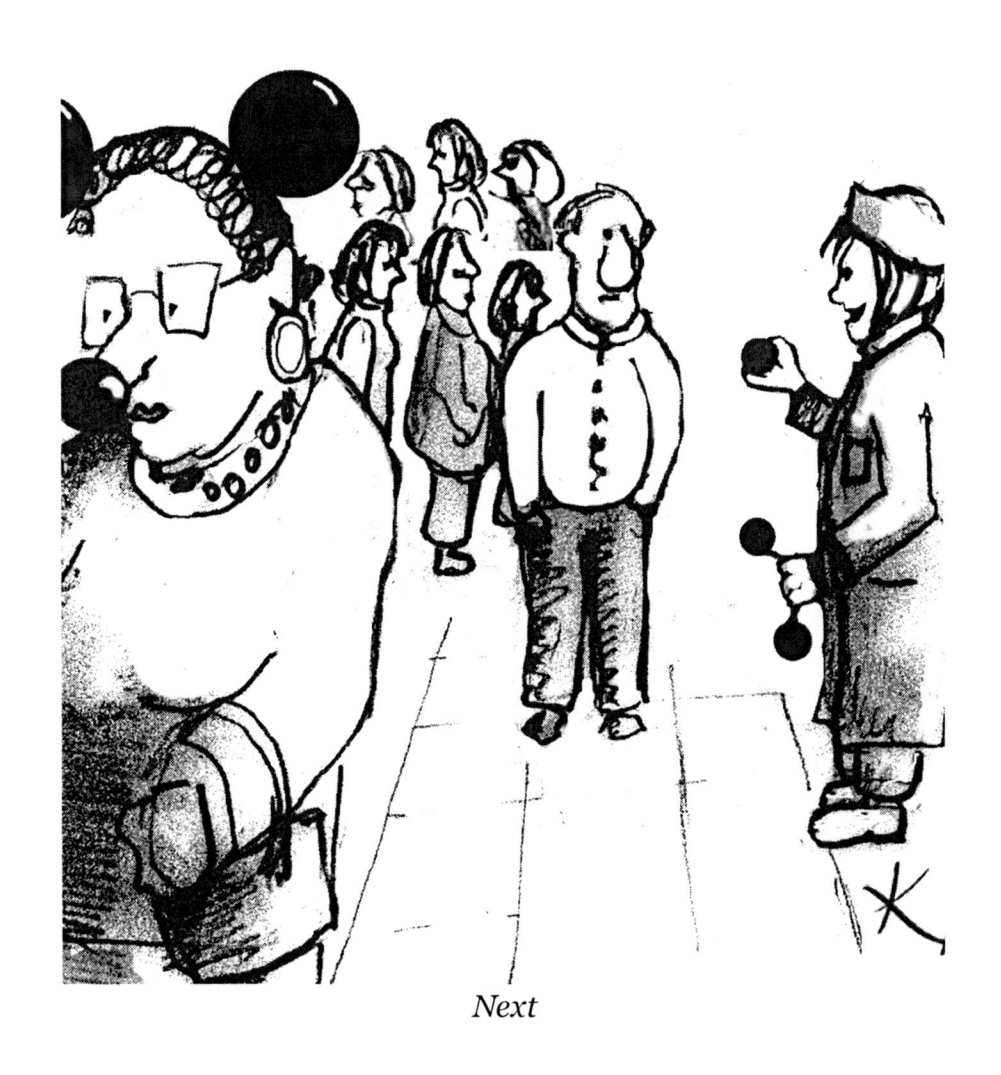

Next

Clinical Trials - Music To Our Ears

The word "clinic" comes from the Greek word *kline*, as in incline. It means couch or bed. Historically, doctors tested their theories by poking and prodding bed-ridden patients to their satisfaction. Today's clinical trials are far more complex and have evolved into four separate stages of experimentation that test new drugs on both healthy and ailing individuals.

Phase 1 trials try to determine how large a dose is both safe and effective. Any new drug has the potential to do more harm than good even though animal testing should have ruled out the possibility of toxic damage to organs. Still, there is always a chance that human tissue will react differently.

Phase 2 trials use a new drug to target a specific medical problem. If the trial is successful it serves as a pilot study that influences the design of larger phase 3 trials.

Phase 3 trials are designed to convince health regulators, like the FDA, to approve the drug for sale to the public. That means demonstrating that the drug is safe and effective.

Phase 4 trials are post-marketing studies that track a drug's performance after it goes on sale.

Less than one molecule in a thousand reaches the level of phase 3 clinical trials. It is a testament to the promise of Acomplia that it is in phase 3 trials on every continent, as a treatment for, not one, but several medical conditions. Here is an outline:

Obesity Trials

Phase 3 trials for Acomplia (its generic name is rimonabant) began in 2001. The largest was the Rimonabant In Obesity program, called RIO for short. The study involved over 3000 participants in North America and another 1500 in Europe. Two additional studies, RIO lipids and RIO Diabetes, enrolled more than 1000 volunteers each.

The RIO trials were designed to show that Acomplia is as safe and effective as a placebo "in conjunction with diet and exercise."[75]

RIO Trial	Status
RIO North America	Complete
RIO Europe	Complete
RIO Lipids	Complete
RIO Diabetes	Complete

Nicotine Addiction

STRATUS (Studies with Rimonabant and Tobacco Use) will test Acomplia as a treatment for nicotine addiction. Three STRATUS programs have been organized: one in the US, one in Europe and one for the rest of the world.

Trial	Status
STRATUS US	Complete
STRATUS EU	Undisclosed
STRATUS World Wide	Undisclosed

Heart Attack and Stroke Trials

These studies are investigating the possibility that Acomplia can reduce heart attacks and stroke among people who are at risk due to their weight.

CRESCENDO was launched in 2005 and will run for 5 years to test the effects of acomplia on the hearts and blood vessels of 17,000 patients.

AUDITOR began its two year run in 2005 while STRADIVARIUS began in early 2006 to see if Acomplia slows down hardening of the arteries.

Trial	Status
CRESCENDO	Incomplete
AUDITOR	Incomplete
STRADIVARIUS	Incomplete

Type 2 Diabetes Trials

SERENADE began in 2005 with 281 participants recently diagnosed with untreated type 2 diabetes to see if Acomplia alone can control blood sugar levels.

ARPEGGIO will evaluate the effect of a daily 20 mg dose of Acomplia on blood glucose levels in type 2 diabetic patients whose insulin treatment is not working as well as it should.

RAPSODI enrolled 2,100 patients in a two-year study that started in 2006 to see if Acomplia can help patients with signs of type 2 diabetes avoid the disease.

Trial	Status
SERENADE	Complete
ARPEGGIO	Incomplete
RAPSODI	Incomplete

These trials involve thousands of volunteers, patients, doctors, technicians and research personnel in the US and thousands more around the globe - including at least one person with an obsession for musical themes.

WHAT'S NEW IN WEIGHT-LOSS DRUGS

*Medicine is a science of uncertainty
and an art of probability.*
~ William Osler

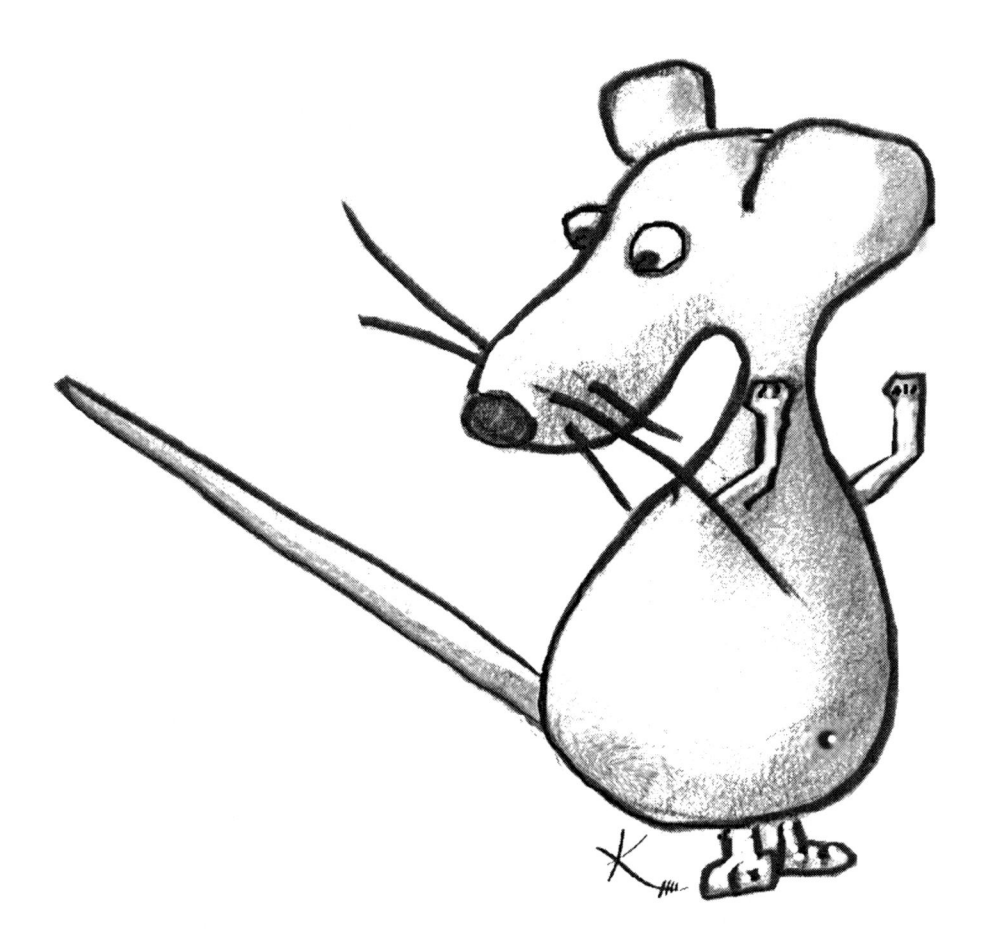

Erectile Dysfunction

Side Effects - The Placebo Factor

Clinical trials are supposed to rule out the possibility of side effects in order to avoid replacing one set of symptoms with another. It's good medicine and good business. Early studies reported that side effects in small mammals were minor. That's promising, but what does that mean for you? Your biology is far more complex and much less predictable.[76]

The animal studies we have seen so far concluded that Acomplia has *no significant side effects*.[77] Is this true? Rodents on a high dose of Acomplia visibly eat less and lose weight, but if they suffer from hidden side effects like nausea, headaches or depression, they aren't saying.

In America, the Food and Drug Administration will not allow drugs to be sold unless they are safe. In general you can be confident that the benefits far outweigh any possible risks, but on an individual basis it's still a gamble when you take medication.

The FDA determines if the risks of taking a drug are acceptable based on data collected during clinical trials. In order for the data to be accurate and meaningful, trials are conducted along strictly scientific lines.

Clinical trials are randomized. If you enroll in a clinical trial, chance determines which treatment you receive. Some patients will get a new drug, some may take an alternative drug and others will receive a placebo. You don't get a choice because the selection process is entirely random.

Placebo

You won't even know which treatment group you are in and neither will your doctor. Trials are double-blinded, which means those receiving the treatment and those who administer it have no idea what is in the medication. Everyone is kept in the dark to avoid contaminating the results.

WHAT'S NEW IN WEIGHT-LOSS DRUGS

As many as half the volunteers who sign up for clinical trials in the hope of finding a remedy could instead be assigned to a placebo. In theory, a placebo helps determine if a new drug works better than nothing at all.

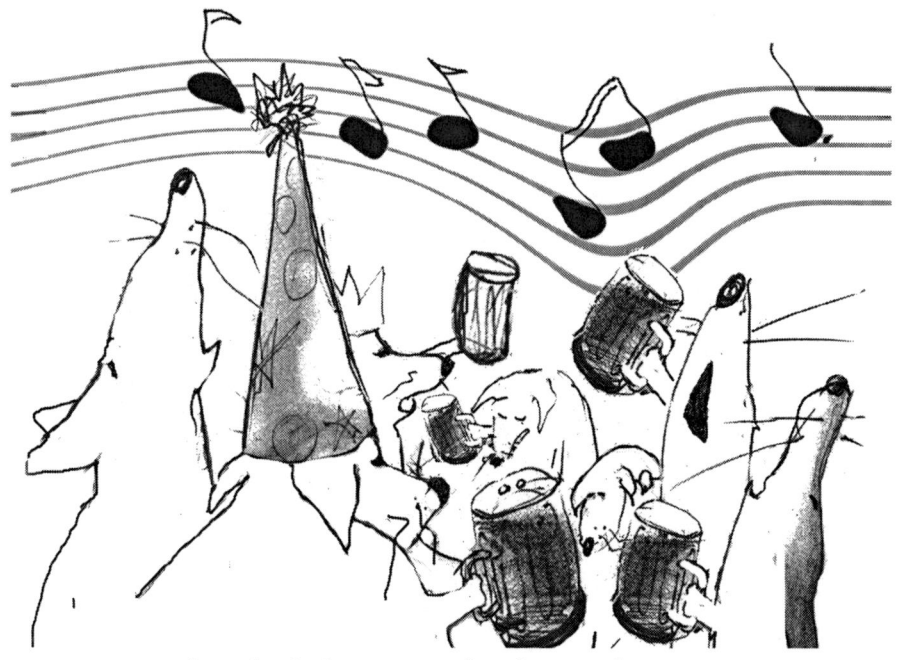

The Alcohol-Versus-Placebo Study Group

Unfortunately, this requires fooling patients into believing they are medicated. Not everyone considers this practice to be helpful or ethical because a patient on a placebo get no effective treatment whatsoever.

The word placebo is Latin for *I will please.* In the past, doctors prescribed a placebo for patients whose symptoms they did not understand or could not treat. Usually, the pill contained an inert substance, often sugar, with no medicinal benefit of any kind.

Denmark is the only western country to allow doctors to prescribe a placebo, maintaining that it does no harm and may even help: the patient is pleased to be treated; the doctor is pleased to be of service; and the chemist is pleased to make a sale. It makes for good feelings all around.

Patients do drop out of clinical trials if they suspect that they have been assigned to a placebo. It's better practice to compare a new drug to *an active comparator*, a drug already on the market that is recognized by experts as the best treatment currently available. In this way, even if you do not receive the experimental drug, you will still benefit from an active medication that has a track record of safety and efficacy.

The difficulty is that good alternatives are sometimes hard to find. Other well known weight-loss drugs are not always effective nor are they free of side effects. Consequently, there was no option but to give half the volunteers in the Acomplia trials a placebo.

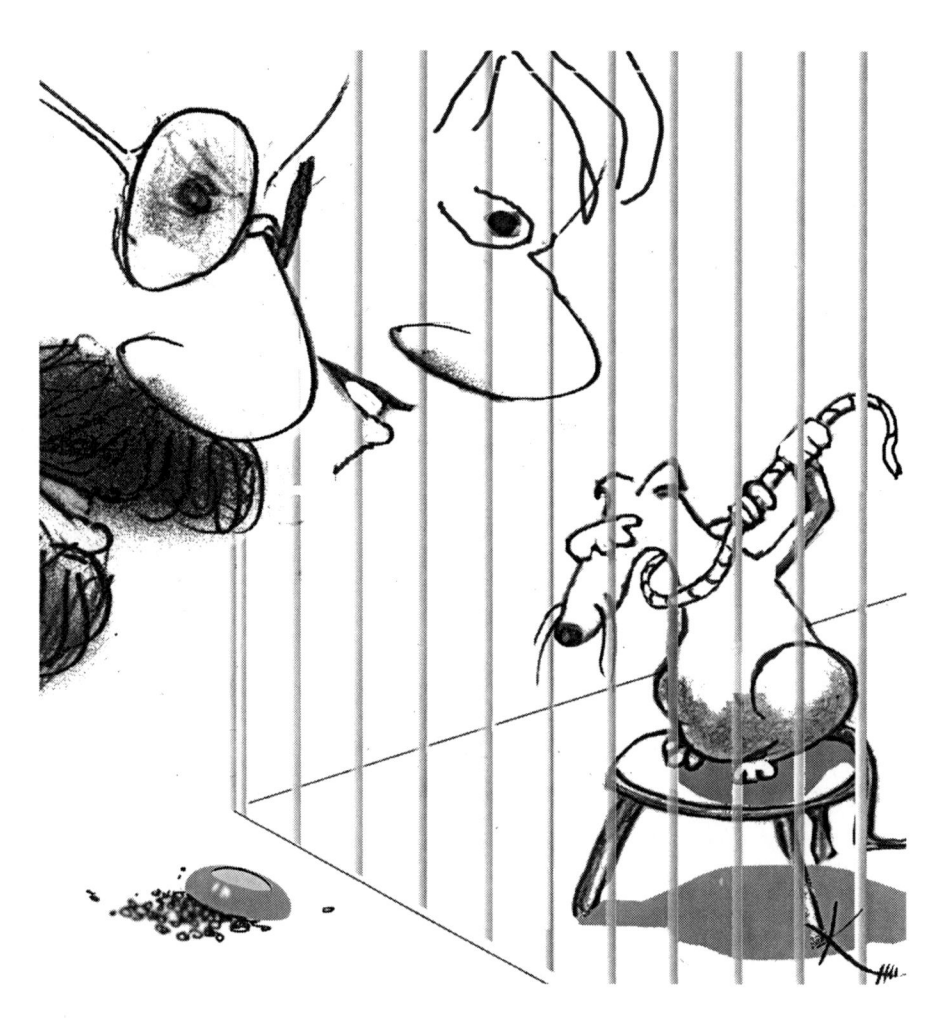

Something tells me he doesn't care for the kibble.

"You can live to be a hundred,
if you give up all the thing that make you want to be a hundred."
~ Woody Allen

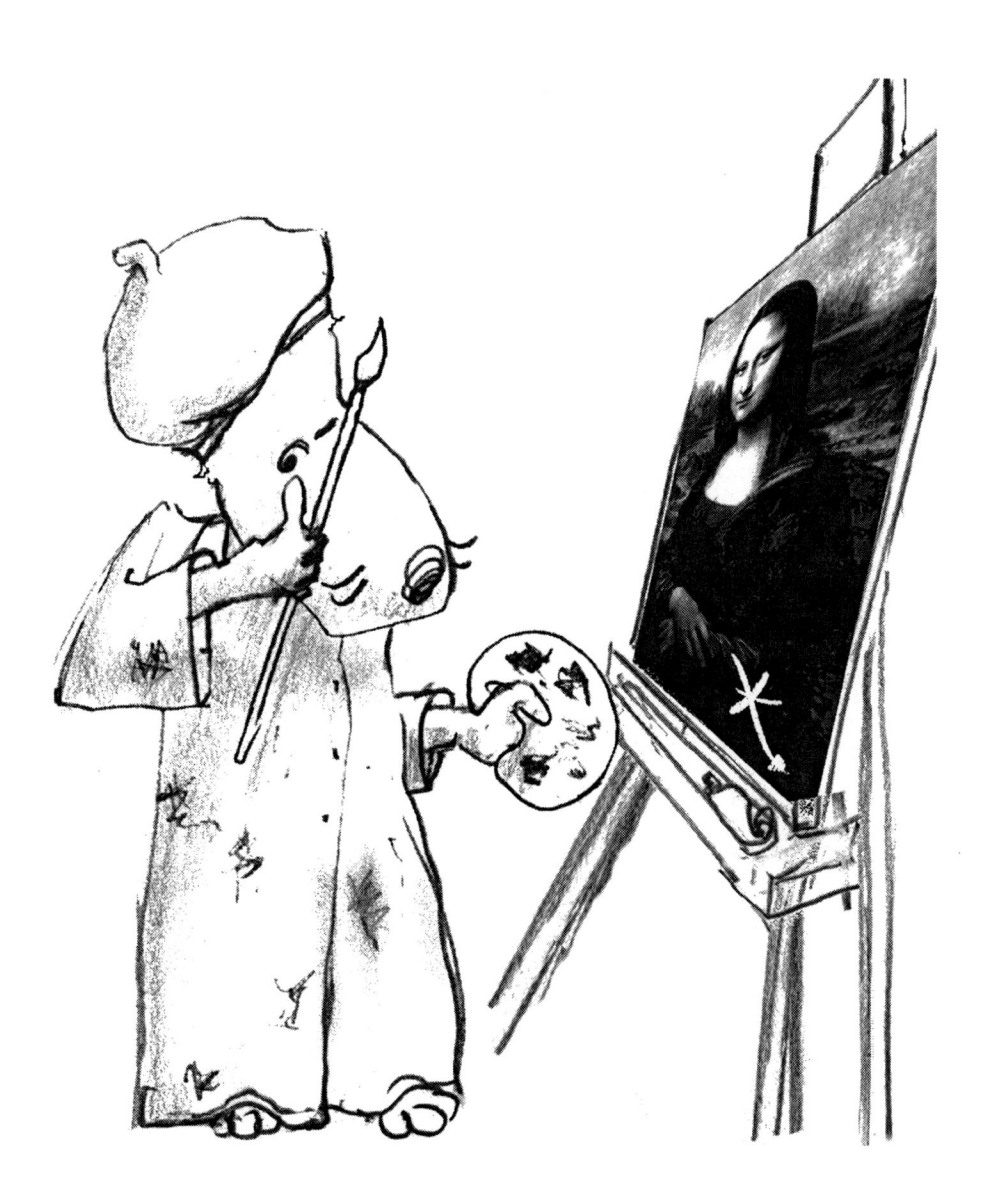

Your Portrait - Painting by Numbers

It's time to look at the results from the RIO North America trial. It might be easier to understand the data if we put a human face on it, especially your face. So let's assume that you are an average volunteer sitting for a statistical portrait.

At the start of the trial you are weighed and measured and cuffed for a blood pressure reading. Then you get to pee in a bottle, get a needle stuck in your arm and have wires glued to your chest. If you have metabolic syndrome, but you're healthy enough to survive the study, you may be an acceptable subject.

Statistically, you are 45 years old. Your odds of being female are five to one. Odds are ten to one you are a non-smoker. You stand 5 feet 4 inches tall in your stockings and your waist measures 42 inches around. You weigh in at 230 pounds and your body mass index is 37.5.

You have elevated levels of sugars and fats floating in your bloodstream and you could be pre-diabetic. Your blood pressure is suspiciously high, but you are not depressed or taking anti-depressants. In brief, you are a white, over weight, middle-age woman who is otherwise healthy and happy-go-lucky.

During the first four weeks of the trial you take a placebo. Everyone does. At the end of this start-up period, you undergo another series of tests to record your vital signs and blood levels. These tests establish a base line marking the departure point for clinical data. From here on, future test results are compared to these numbers.

Next, everyone is randomly assigned to one of three treatment groups. The smallest group of 607 patients receives a placebo from start to finish. A group of 1216 patients receive a low dose (5 mg/day) of Acomplia. You are in the last group of 1222 patients who receive a high daily dose (20 mg/day) of Acomplia.

What you do not suspect is that your group will be randomized again after one year. Half of you will unknowingly switch to a placebo to determine how long Acomplia continues to be effective after treatment stops. Your group will continue taking Acomplia until the end.

For the next two years, you eat sensibly and work out regularly. You report for scheduled interviews to prove that you are still alive and kicking. You have regular checkups, more heart and blood tests and an opportunity to share any medical or personal concerns with your doctor, particularly if you are experiencing side effects.

After two years you lose 14 pounds, about 6% of your body mass. A few individuals lose as much as 20 pounds. The average weight loss in the placebo group is only 5 pounds. Your waistline shrank by 3 inches while the placebo group lost less than one inch.

Typical blood pressure for healthy adults is 120 over 80 while at rest. At baseline, yours was 122 over 78. By the end of the trial, Acomplia had lowered your blood pressure only slightly.

Acomplia had its most dramatic effect on your blood chemistry. HDL cholesterol, the good kind, increased by 9.5% compared to the placebo group. LDL cholesterol, the bad kind, did not decrease significantly, but your triglyceride levels are down 7.4% compared to the placebo average.[78] This means you are storing less fat, breaking it down and flushing it away.

You experienced some nausea and an occasional bout of depression during the first year, but you have lost weight, feel better and look healthier than you did two years ago.

Medically speaking, your vital signs are strong and your body chemistry is headed in a healthy direction. Your metabolism is dealing more efficiently with fats and sugars and your risk of heart attack and diabetes is reduced substantially.

You are still officially over weight, but otherwise you are a statistical picture of health.

*"I used to eat a lot of natural foods
until I learned that most people die of natural causes."
~ Unknown*

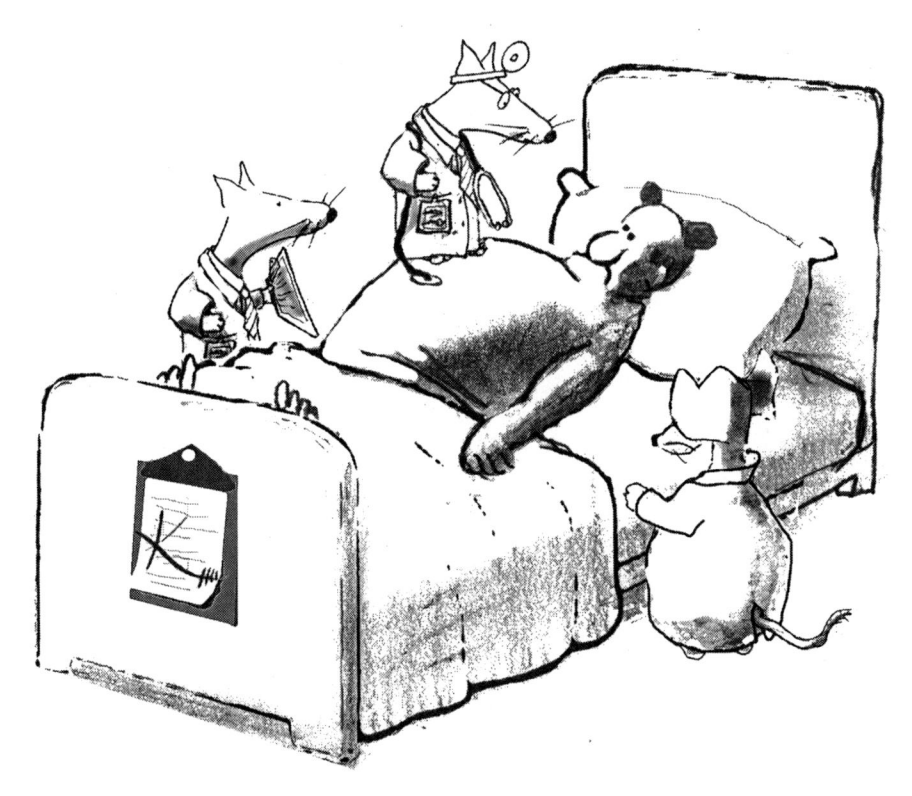

Animal Studies

Acomplia – Is It For You?

Statistically speaking, Acomplia does what it is supposed to do: it reduces body weight and waist size and improves blood chemistry. But realistically, each of us is very different. Until you take Acomplia yourself, you won't know what effect the drug has on you or what effect you will have on the drug.

There are other factors to consider as well. In addition to taking Acomplia, North American volunteers changed their eating habits and exercised regularly. In other words, they abruptly altered the pattern of their lives.

The question is, how can the effects of Acomplia be properly measured with so many changes occurring at the same time.[79] How do you know for certain what causes either a side effect or a benefit?

Diet and exercise together can be very effective at reducing weight and improving cholesterol levels. In fact, it was diet and exercise, not Acomplia, that reduced everyone's risk factors during the four week start-up period when all participants took a placebo.

Among those who stayed on Acomplia for the entire two years, this brief placebo period was responsible for more than 25% of their weight loss, 25% of their reduction in waist size and significantly lower triglyceride levels.

Acomplia helped maintain and increase weight loss, but the data does not reveal how much of the credit should go to Acomplia, to diet or to exercise. We don't really know what Acomplia can achieve on its own.

Furthermore, most of the volunteers in the American RIO trial were white, middle-aged women classified as morbidly obese. If you do not fit into that category, these trial results may not apply to you at all.

Is Acomplia Safe?

When Sanofi-Aventis sought approval for Acomplia as a weight loss drug in 2006 the FDA turned them down – and then again in 2007. Does this mean that Acomplia is dangerous?

Any new drug must be less harmful than the disorder it is treating. For Acomplia, that was a problem because obesity (never mind weight gain) is not officially recognized as a medical condition. A strict interpretation would find that there is no disease and therefore Acomplia must be completely harmless.

The case for Acomplia was weakened by data showing it to be less safe than a placebo by a few percentage points. In other words, Acomplia is more dangerous than doing nothing.

A bigger concern is that 55% of those patients who successfully lost weight on Acomplia still decided to drop out of the trial. You may find that alarming, so let's put that number in perspective.

First, as many as half the participants in weight related clinical trials leave for one reason or another. That is not unusual. Second, although 85% of patients on a high dose of Acomplia reported uncomfortable side effects, 82% of patients taking a placebo experienced the same discomfort.

Roughly 24% of drop-outs said that adverse effects were the main reason for leaving. Nausea was the most common complaint, followed by depression and anxiety.

By the end of the trial, almost 1900 patients dropped out of the program. About 40% officially requested to leave and 15% quit without notification. Approximately 10% abandoned the study because they saw no improvement.

When you take all this into account, the drop-out rate for Acomplia is less dramatic. Still, you are statistically more likely to experience side effects with Acomplia than with a placebo.

Sanofi-Aventis maintains that the drop-out rate was consistent with previous studies in over weight patients, but no matter how you add it up, Acomplia still caused more drop-outs due to depression than a placebo.[80]

Unlike obesity, depression is a recognized disease with dangerous and sometimes immediate consequences. Acomplia is suspect because it affects the brain's pleasure centers, but that does not explain why almost as many placebo patients had the same problem

Is Acomplia Worth the Risks?

Will Acomplia make you depressed? It's possible. It is also possible that if you exercise moderately and eat sensibly for two years and take 20 mg of Acomplia every day you can drop a few pounds, lose a few inches around your middle and improve your chances of avoiding a heart attack and diabetes.

If you are desperately over weight you might be tempted to try Acomplia. With luck, you may experience none of the usual side effects, but that does not mean you are safe.

WHAT'S NEW IN WEIGHT-LOSS DRUGS

One immediate problem is the danger posed by purchasing Acomplia online. Be aware that you have no guarantees that the medications you illegally import into the US are either safe or effective.

As for side effects, some drugs have been linked to organ failure years after they were approved. Just because no long-term side effects have shown up yet doesn't mean there aren't any.

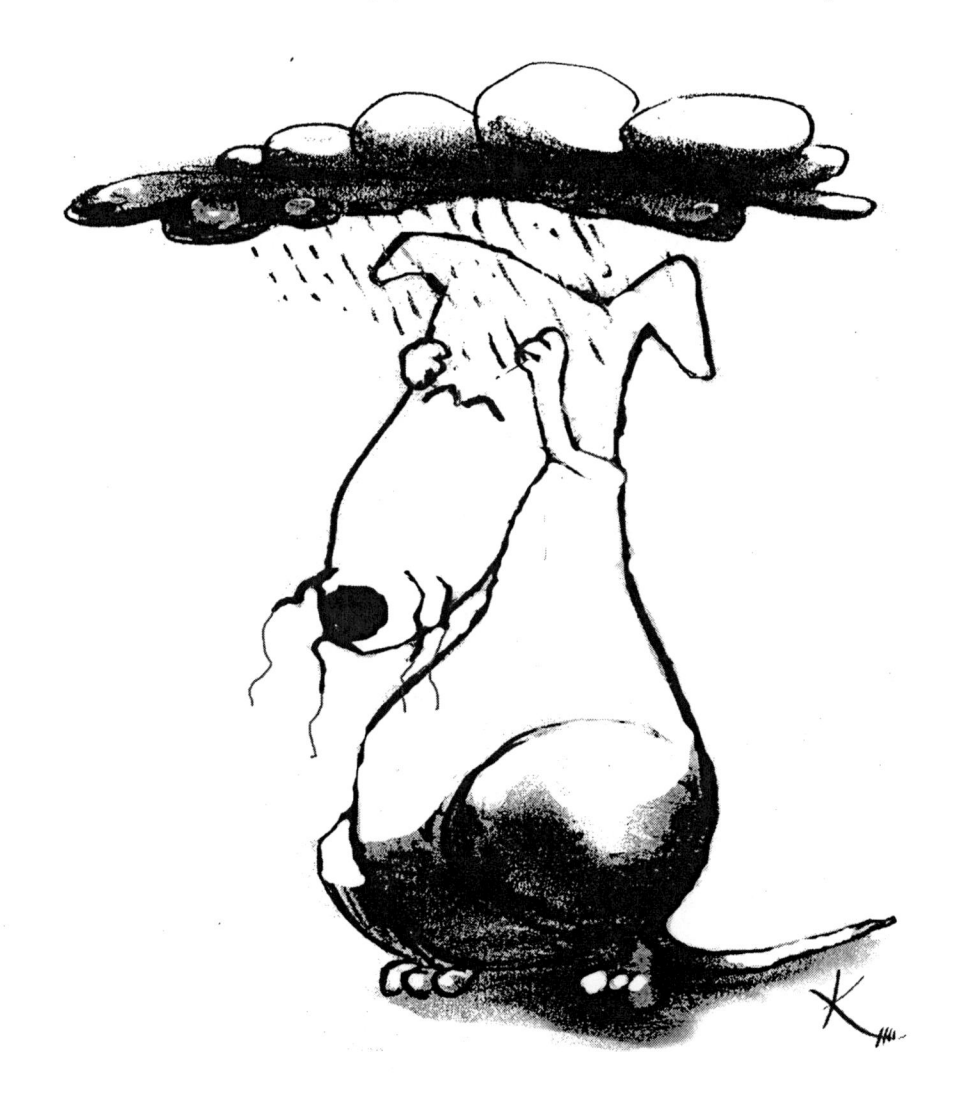

> "Everything I eat
> has been proved by some doctor or other
> to be a deadly poison,
> and everything I don't eat
> has been proved to be indispensable for life."
> ~ George Bernard Shaw
> (1856–1950)

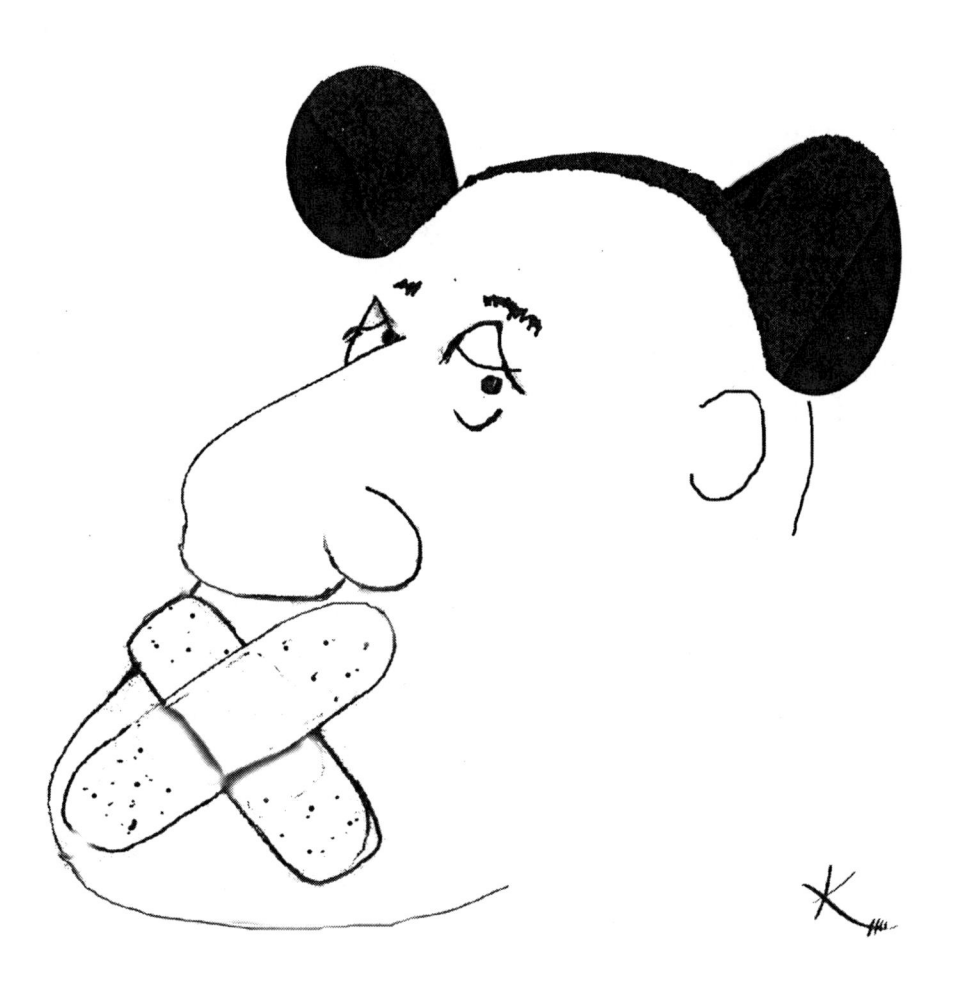

Acomplia and Diabetes

Your brain depends on insulin signaling to monitor your energy needs. Insulin is a hormone that breaks down sugar into glucose to make energy. Without it, you can't meet your energy requirements.

When you have type 1 diabetes, the cells that produce insulin are damaged or destroyed. When you have type 2 diabetes, insulin is available, but your body ignores it – a condition known as insulin resistance. Excess sugar in your blood and a surplus of fat on your body could be signs of insulin resistance.

While the FDA denied approval to Acomplia as a weight loss medication, it's possible that Acomplia will eventually be approved for the treatment and prevention of diabetes. Acomplia produced some impressive results during its RIO-diabetes trial.[81] The trial lasted for one year and involved more than 1000 volunteers from eleven European countries.

In this study, patients ate a low calorie diet, but they were not expected to exercise. Men and women were equally represented, they averaged 56 years of age and were over weight with high blood sugar levels and other symptoms of diabetes.

A high dose (20mg) of Acomplia obtained good results compared to a placebo. The average weight loss was 12 pounds, about four times the placebo rate. On average, waists shrank 2 inches, three times the placebo rate. Healthy HDL-cholesterol levels were twice as high for Acomplia compared to a placebo. Triglycerides dropped more than 9% with Acomplia while rising more than 7% with a placebo.

Among those patients who were already diabetic, Acomplia lowered blood sugar levels below the 6.5% target set by the American Diabetes Association. Only one quarter of the placebo group achieved as much.

WHAT'S NEW IN WEIGHT-LOSS DRUGS

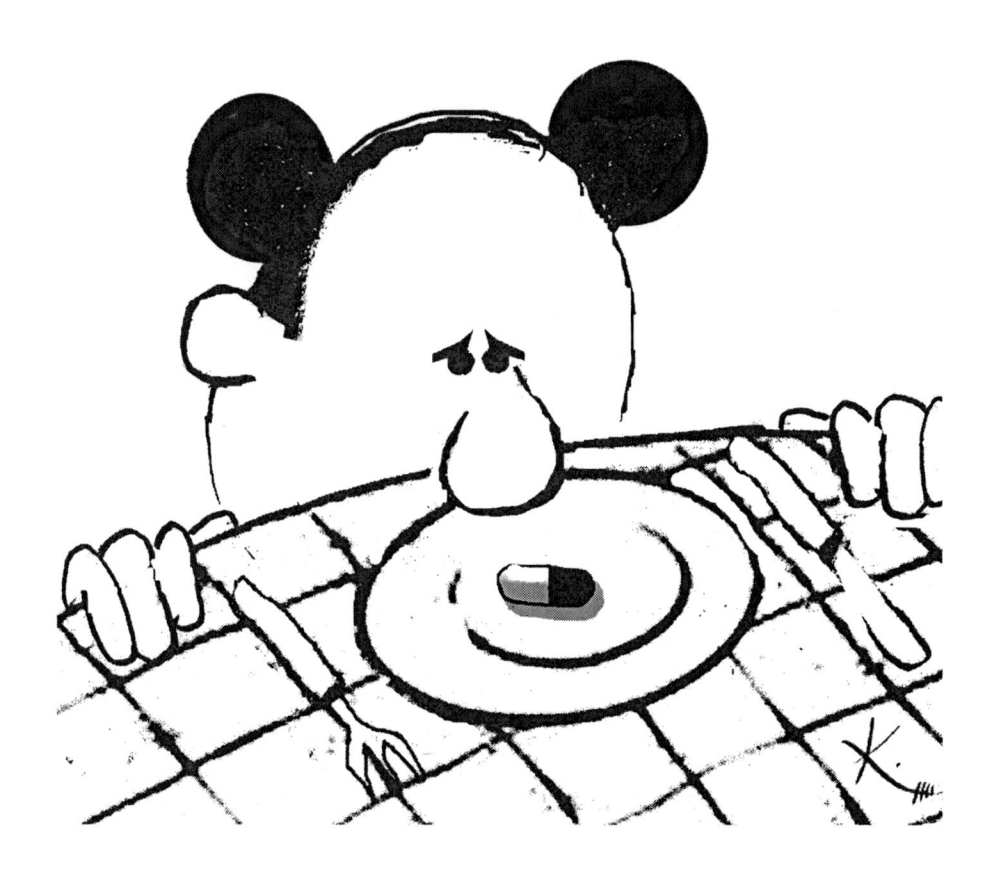

Acomplia also improved lipid profiles, so much so that 20% of patients were no longer considered to have metabolic syndrome. That was 2.5 times more than the placebo group.

Acomplia was also responsible for more than half the improvement in blood sugar levels and it had twice the impact on HDL-cholesterol, triglycerides, fasting insulin and insulin sensitivity than can be explained by weight loss alone.

The RIO results were supported by a smaller, 6 month long trial called SERENADE, where 278 people with type 2 diabetes put Acomplia through its paces.

Patients on Acomplia lost almost 15 pounds while the placebo group lost less than 6 pounds; their waist line shrank by 2.34 inches compared to less than an inch; and their blood sugar level decreased 1.9 points compared to 0.7 points.

Good cholesterol increased by 10.1% compared to 3.2% in the placebo group. Triglyceride levels went down 16.3% versus 4.4%. Adiponectin went up while fasting blood sugar levels dropped.

Again, the improvement in blood sugar levels (57%) could not be explained by weight-loss alone which points to Acomplia as the source of additional benefits.

In both studies, Acomplia patients experienced more side effects than those on a placebo. Nausea, upper respiratory infection, depression and headache were the main complaints.

Again, the majority of drop-outs came from the Acomplia group. That should not alarm you. You may still benefit from Acomplia. Some diabetics take medications that cause potentially dangerous weight gain. It's a matter of judging your risks versus the benefits in consultation with your doctor.

The lesson here is that no drug is perfect. Acomplia is not for everyone, but it is fair to say that many individuals did benefit from taking Acomplia. Some of them lost weight and experienced only mild side effects or none at all.

WHAT'S NEW IN WEIGHT-LOSS DRUGS

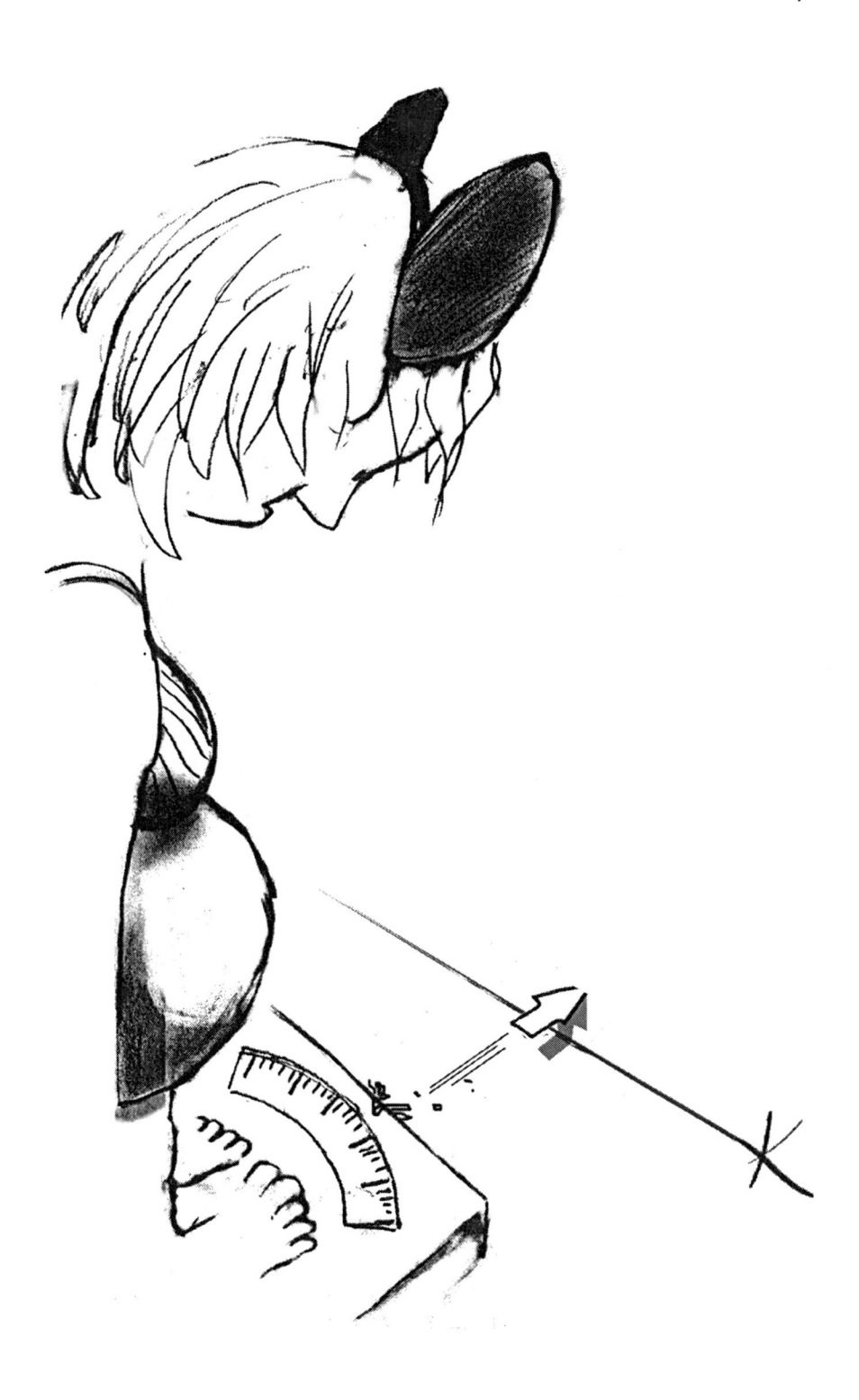

PART FOUR

FUTURE CONSIDERATIONS

*"When I read about the evils of drinking,
I gave up reading."
~ Henny Youngman*

WHAT'S NEW IN WEIGHT-LOSS DRUGS   121

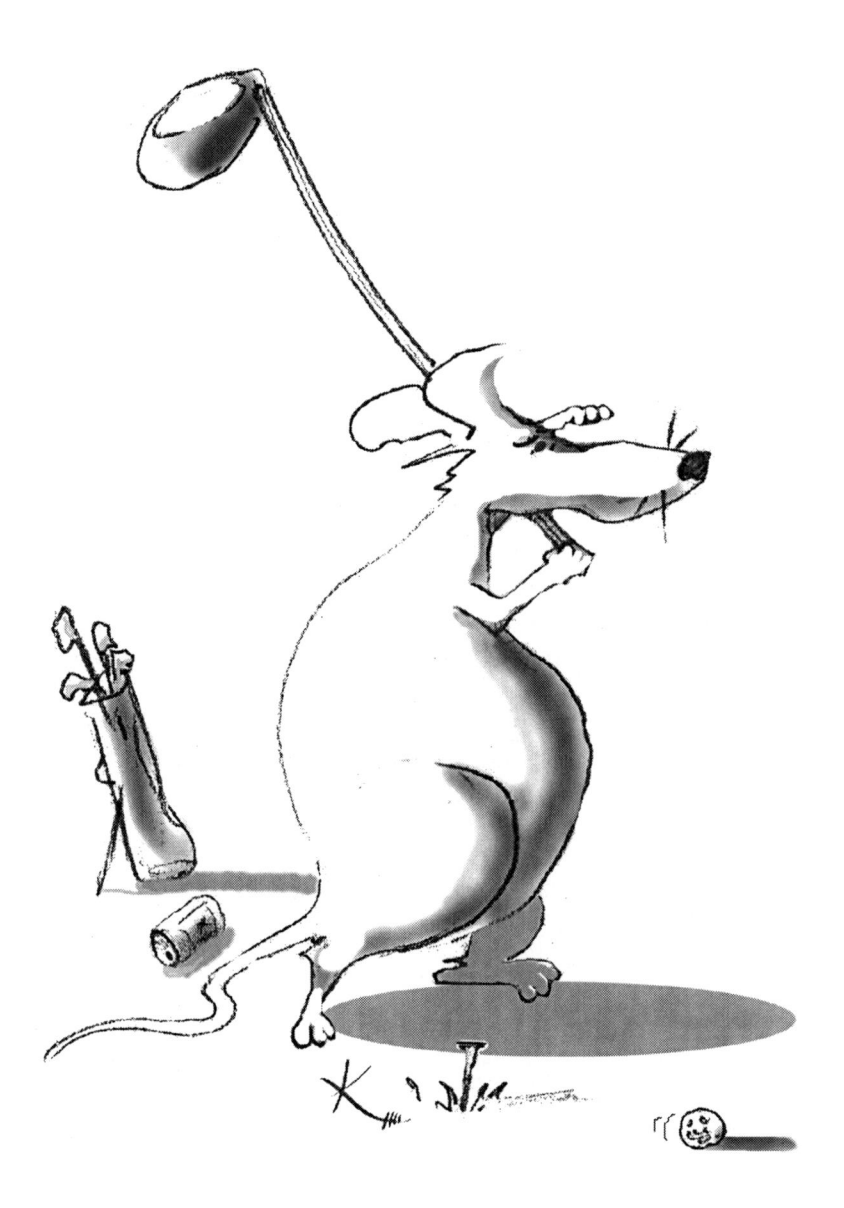

Alcohol – Rats That Drink and Drive

About two billion people around the world drink alcohol, so when the National Institute on Alcohol Abuse and Alcoholism (NIAAA) launched a study of Acomplia and alcoholism in 2003, there was no shortage of volunteers.[82]

Millions of Americans are alcohol dependent and millions more suffer from alcohol-related injuries, alcohol-induced cancers, chronic diseases and family breakups. Experts say that the financial cost of alcohol abuse in America approaches $200 billion when treatment, lost productivity and policing are included.

And yet alcohol remains a popular and legal commodity, one we associate with good times and fellowship. We conveniently forget that alcohol is toxic and addicting.

Every now and then another study reveals that moderate alcohol consumption is beneficial because it lowers blood pressure and reduces the risk of heart attack and stroke. Resveratrol, for example, is a compound found in red wine that extends the life span of rodents. You would have to drink red wine all day, every day to gain a similar advantage.

You may also have heard that nicotine is sometimes beneficial because it reduces stress and controls over-eating. There is some truth in this, but the damage done by alcohol or nicotine far outweighs any benefits. Otherwise, your doctor would prescribe a cheeky Merlot and a pack of smokes for hypertension!

Have you noticed how booze and cigarettes seem to go together? There is a good reason for this. Researchers at Texas A&M report that "cigarette smoking appears to promote the consumption of alcohol".[83]

They found that rats that drink and smoke have half as much alcohol in their blood stream as non-smokers. This suggests that smokers need to drink twice as much as non-smokers to get the same buzz.

In theory, you might expect a stimulant like nicotine to negate the mood-altering effects of a depressant like alcohol, and vice versa, but that is not what happens. Smoking and drinking at the same time provide more pleasure than either one alone because they both promote dopamine release.

Alcohol makes you feel good, temporarily, but it depresses your central nervous system which slows down neural signaling. Over time it changes your brain chemistry and disturbs the balance between two opposing chemicals: glutamate and GABA.

Glutamate is the most common neurotransmitter in the brain. It appears to strengthen communications between nerve cells that regularly share messages by helping receptors to grow where they are most needed.

GABA (gamma-aminobutyric acid) slows down signaling. This is a critical function, especially when receptors are bombarded so relentlessly by incoming messenger molecules that they are in danger of burning out.

Alcohol is sedating because it simultaneously eases up on the gas pedal (glutamate) and pushes down on the brake pedal (GABA). This sudden loss of brain activity is the celebrated condition known as intoxication.

The occasional drink, like the occasional cigarette, may seem harmless enough, but they both have immediate effects on your brain. Casual drinkers consider the trade-off between risk and pleasure to be worthwhile - the pleasure being almost immediate whereas the consequences are delayed.

Your sensitivity to alcohol probably depends on your genes and the number of GABA receptors you have.[84] If you are a regular drinker, you run the risk of desensitizing your GABA receptors to the point where increasingly more alcohol is needed to achieve the same level of pleasure. If you tolerate alcohol, then you can drink as much as you need to take some pleasure from it.

The trouble is, the more you drink, the more damage you do. In time, alcohol changes the surface of your brain cells (not to mention your liver) causing permanent injury and tissue degeneration.[85] Symptoms include a weak memory, loss of motor control, variations in body temperature, insensitivity to pain and a lack of energy.

So what has all this to do with Acomplia? If you look at a map of alcohol-related brain damage in humans you will see that it neatly corresponds with the distribution of CB1 receptors. That suggests that the effects of alcohol probably depend on CB1 receptors. In that case, Acomplia could be protective against intoxication or alcoholism.

Evidence for this lies in the fact that elderly mice do not drink alcohol.[86] It has nothing to do with being older and wiser. When researchers found that Acomplia failed to reduce hunger in older mice, they accidentally discovered that aging mice have a shortage of healthy, new CB1 receptors. Old mice lose interest in alcohol because their CB1 receptors wear out. It explains why Acomplia has little or no effect on their appetite.

CB1 receptors are essential to the appreciation of alcoholic drinks. We know this because CB1 knockout mice prefer water to alcohol. Studies with rodents of all stripes, be they abstainers, social drinkers or alcoholics, show that alcohol abuse is definitely linked to CB1 receptors.[87-88]

Acomplia can reduce heavy drinking temporarily, but mice that drink have more active CB1 receptors than non-drinkers and sooner or later, they start craving alcohol again.[89]

Alcohol gradually loses its ability to lift your mood because CB1 receptors get tuckered out. Alcohol makes matters worse obstructing the genes responsible for growing new CB1 receptors, especially in the midbrain. As a result, loose cannabinoids find other receptors to bind to in your forebrain. From there, they can operate as an incentive to drink more by eroding your normal inhibitions and suspending rational judgment.

Alcohol also interferes with the activity of enzymes that promote healing and replacement of damaged receptors. Adenylate cyclase (AC), for example, is unable to do its job of building new messenger molecules. Without them, neural signals become weaker. Brain cells are unable to respond to incoming hormones and they fail to initiate repairs or adapt to changing conditions.

In test tube experiments, individual brain cells become tolerant to alcohol and dependent on it within 72 hours of exposure. As the cells adapt to alcohol, they increasingly over-activate an enzyme called phospholipase (PLA2) that manufactures cannabinoids.[90]

That leads to a vicious cycle where an excess of alcohol damages CB1 receptors but triggers the over-production of cannabinoids that trigger more drinking … and so on.

Rats that drink heavily produce as many cannabinoids as rats who suffer brain injuries severe enough to cause tissue degeneration and death. Chemically speaking, there is little difference between heavy drinking and banging your head against a wall.

Rats genuinely enjoy beer and sometimes drink to excess.[91] In one experiment, rats had access to an open bar where one lick at a tap released one drop of beer. Then, the price of beer went up - two licks earned one drop. Then three. As the cost kept climbing, the number of licks increased to the point that even thirsty rats gave up drinking.[92]

You can measure the motivation to drink by counting the number of licks a rat is prepared to make before it hits the break point and quits. In several experiments, the break point was pushed higher by stimulating the CB1 receptors. Stronger doses of stimulant moved the break point higher still. There is a clear link between the activation of CB1 receptors and the motivation to drink.

WHAT'S NEW IN WEIGHT-LOSS DRUGS   127

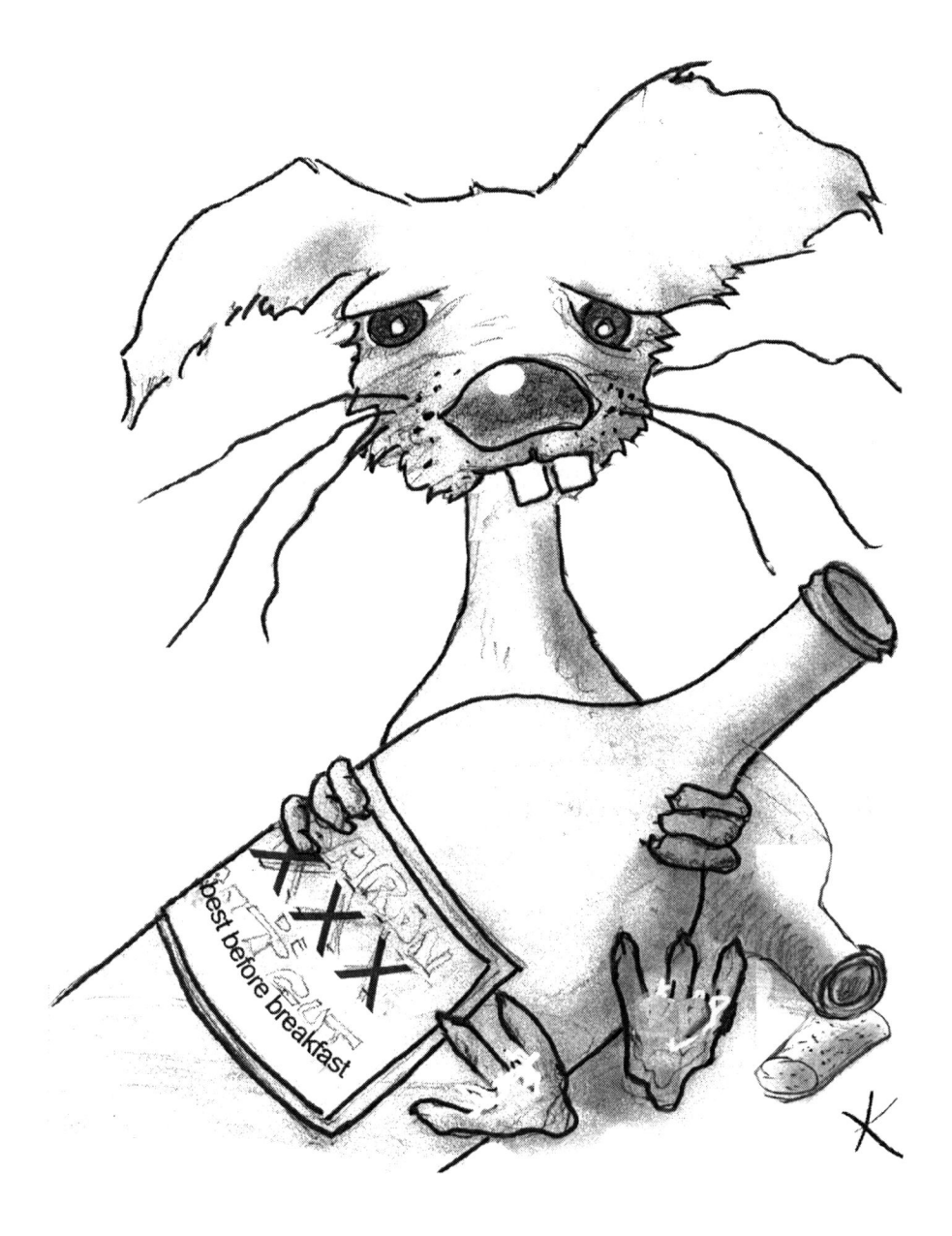

When the same rats took Acomplia, the break point fell dramatically. As with food, Acomplia reversed alcohol intake significantly, but not completely. That's because CB1 receptors do not work alone.

Once again, opioid receptors play a role, this time to motivate alcohol consumption. Together, active CB1 and opioid receptors overpower Acomplia and bring our rats back to the bar.

But that is not the end of the story. There is a breed of dedicated drinkers called Sardinian alcohol-preferring rats. They drink other rats under the table. Stimulate their receptors and they drink more still.

Inexplicably, Acomplia virtually eliminates drinking behavior in these rats.[93] It remains a mystery how a small dose of Acomplia could have such an impact when the odds are firmly against it.[94]

The implications for human treatment are obvious and there is a growing interest in Acomplia as experiments continue to demonstrate its remarkable ability to reduce alcohol intake.[95] In December of 2003, the National Institute on Alcohol Abuse and Alcoholism launched a US study to assess the safety and efficacy of Acomplia as a treatment for alcoholism.[96] No trial results have yet been posted.

Cheers!

"I make it a rule never to smoke while I'm sleeping."
~ Mark Twain

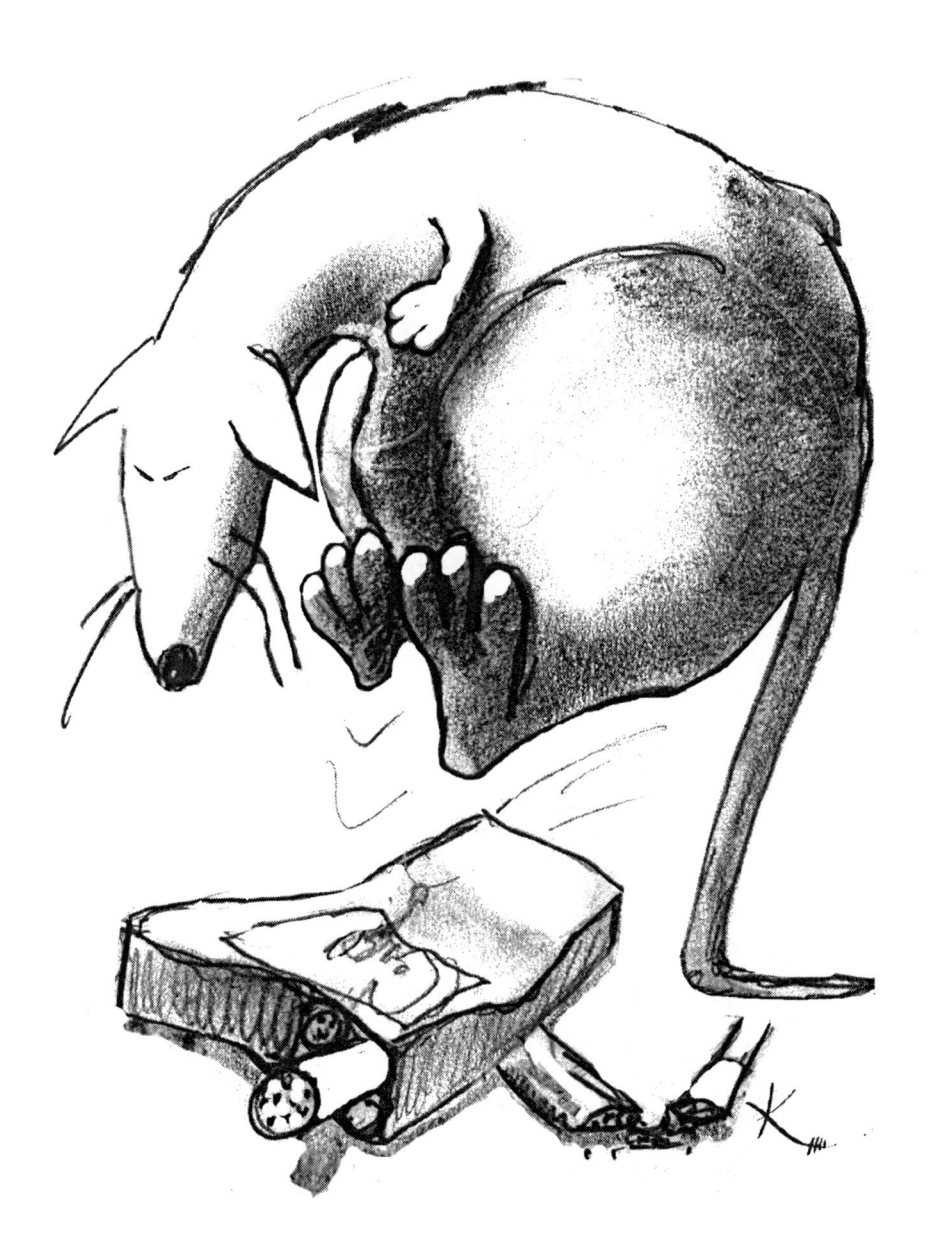

Nicotine – Furry Quitters

Some rats smoke the human equivalent of a pack of cigarettes a day. They enjoy nicotine for the same reason they enjoy alcohol or sweets – it stimulates dopamine release.

Nicotine is especially effective at raising dopamine levels because it over-activates the cannabinoid system.[97] Rats smoke more frequently when their CB1 receptors are excited and the more they smoke, the more they want to smoke.

Numerous experiments have demonstrated that Acomplia reduces smoking, but one experiment involving rats stands out from the rest because it shows us how seductive nicotine can be.[98]

Rats with regular access to cigarette smoke, found themselves whisked off to a special room whenever they inhaled. The room had a floor made of narrow bars that made it difficult to relax. In that place, the uncomfortable place, the rats experienced the effects of nicotine.

At first, most rats preferred to sit in an adjacent room where a comfortable mesh floor made sitting or standing much easier. As their addiction grew, they increasingly spent more time in the designated smoking area - much like humans huddled in the doorways of wind-blown office towers during cigarette breaks.

Despite the physical discomfort, these rats considered the smoking room to be a *feel good* place. They had made a connection between their environment and the effects of nicotine.

In contrast, rats treated with Acomplia did not display the same behavior. They appeared to enjoy nicotine, but they did not crave it or seek it. The uncomfortable room had no special appeal for them.

WHAT'S NEW IN WEIGHT-LOSS DRUGS

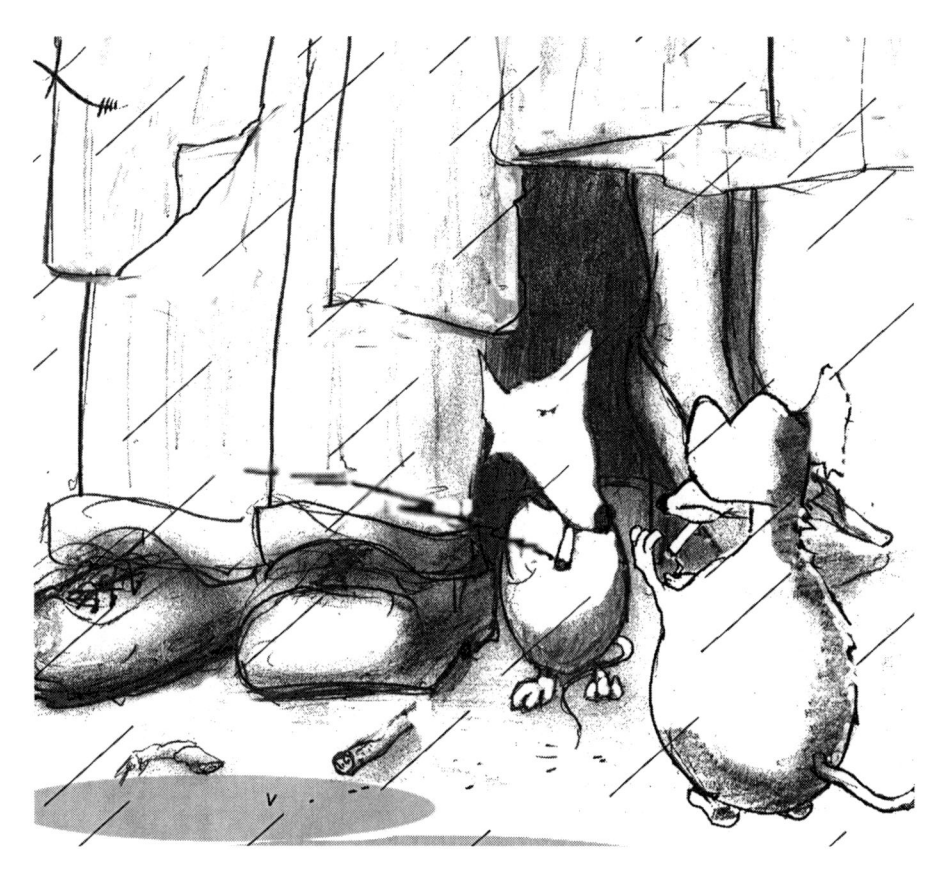

Coffee Break at the Lab

Rats taking Acomplia inhaled just as much nicotine, but they did not make the same connection possibly because Acomplia reduced the production of dopamine. Without sufficient dopamine, these rats were either unable to learn or unable to remember that the pleasure of nicotine was linked to a specific location.

Memories induced by nicotine are so strong that only very high doses of Acomplia can break the connection.[99] Nicotine creates such enduring memories that they persist long after symptoms of withdrawal have disappeared.

There is a good example of this. Smoking rats that learned to press a lever for nicotine also triggered feedback in the form of light and sound whenever they did so.[100] One day, the nicotine supply was cut off. Pressing the lever turned on the light and made a noise, but no rewarding nicotine arrived.

The rats were so conditioned to the association between nicotine and the audio-visual display that they continued to press the lever for another three months. Even a large dose of Acomplia failed to slow them down. In the end, the elimination of all feedback put a stop to lever pressing.

Nicotine memories make it very difficult for humans to quit smoking too. They need to overcome nicotine-induced expectations, but that won't be easy. Among the unidentified toxins and unknown substances in cigarette smoke is a chemical that prevents the break down of dopamine. The enzyme that usually does that job is blocked and as a result, dopamine lingers in the brain, entrenching nicotine memories.

Compounding the problem, nicotine raises dopamine levels itself by turning on acetylcholine receptors. Acetylcholine (AC) was the first and the most common neurotransmitter found in the human nervous system. Your parasympathetic nervous system, which governs every breath you take, is entirely dependent on signals from AC receptors.

Some AC receptors are so hospitable to nicotine that they have earned the name nicotinic receptors. When they are turned on, they communicate with the nucleus accumbens and trigger dopamine release.

Although nicotine is addictive and potentially deadly, the cigarette break is still a popular form of reward seeking, a chance to settle the nerves and clear the mind. It's dopamine that provides the heightened sense of awareness and sense of well-being that provides so much satisfaction.

Unfortunately, cigarettes lose their rewarding properties over time because receptors gradually become tolerant or weaken from constant demand. More nicotine, more often, is required to spark a minimal hint of pleasure.

If you attempt to quit smoking, you can expect to meet physical and psychological resistance as your body and mind attempt to subvert your will power. As you sleep, your receptors regain some of their sensitivity. When you wake up in the morning after eight hours of nicotine withdrawal, your acetylcholine levels have risen dramatically and literally leave you itching for a smoke.

If you want to quit, your options are limited.[101] Smokers spend in excess of $350 billion annually on nicotine patches, gums and sprays searching for some form of nicotine substitute. Roughly 70% of them start smoking again.

Finding a new nicotine treatment is a medical priority. Ideally, any drug that reduces cigarette smoking should control your cravings and gently restore acetylcholine levels to avoid withdrawal symptoms. It should reduce stress, control hunger, prevent weight gain, erase memories of nicotine euphoria and make it possible to leap tall buildings in a single bound!

That's a lot to ask and so far, that drug does not exist. If you have tried to quit smoking with the help of your doctor, you may have taken Welbutrin, also known as Bupropion. This is an anti-depressant and the only drug to earn approval from the FDA for smoking cessation. It is not clear why it helps some people and not others.[102-103]

If you plan to quit smoking in the future, here are three noteworthy solutions currently in the works.

Varenicline is a new drug still in development that looks promising because it works directly on the nicotinic receptors.[104] Hopefully, it will moderate dopamine release and control chemical dependency.

Another solution may come in the form of nicotine vaccines like NicVAX, which has been in clinical trials since early in 2006.[105] Vaccines stimulates antibodies that protect the brain from nicotine by limiting the production of dopamine. They have few side effects and work reasonably well, depending on the individual, but so far, they wear off in a day or so.

In March of 2004, Dr. Robert Anthenelli suggested another solution to the American College of Cardiology.[106] He had just concluded a ten-week trial of 787 American patients who wanted to quit smoking with the help of an experimental drug.

Most of his patients had smoked a pack of cigarettes a day for up to 24 years. All of them had tried and failed to quit in the past. According to his data, this new drug doubled their chances of quitting.

Remarkably, over one third of his patients lost weight after they quit and they experienced no serious side effects. Patients who took the drug for up to a year lost 5% of their body weight without a change of diet or an increase in exercise.

The name of this new drug was, of course, Acomplia. The FDA requested more trial data before granting approval as a treatment for smoking-cessation, but Sanofi-Aventis has indicated no interest in pursuing the matter at this time.

*"A drug is a substance given to rats
to produce a scientific paper."*
~ Unknown

WHAT'S NEW IN WEIGHT-LOSS DRUGS

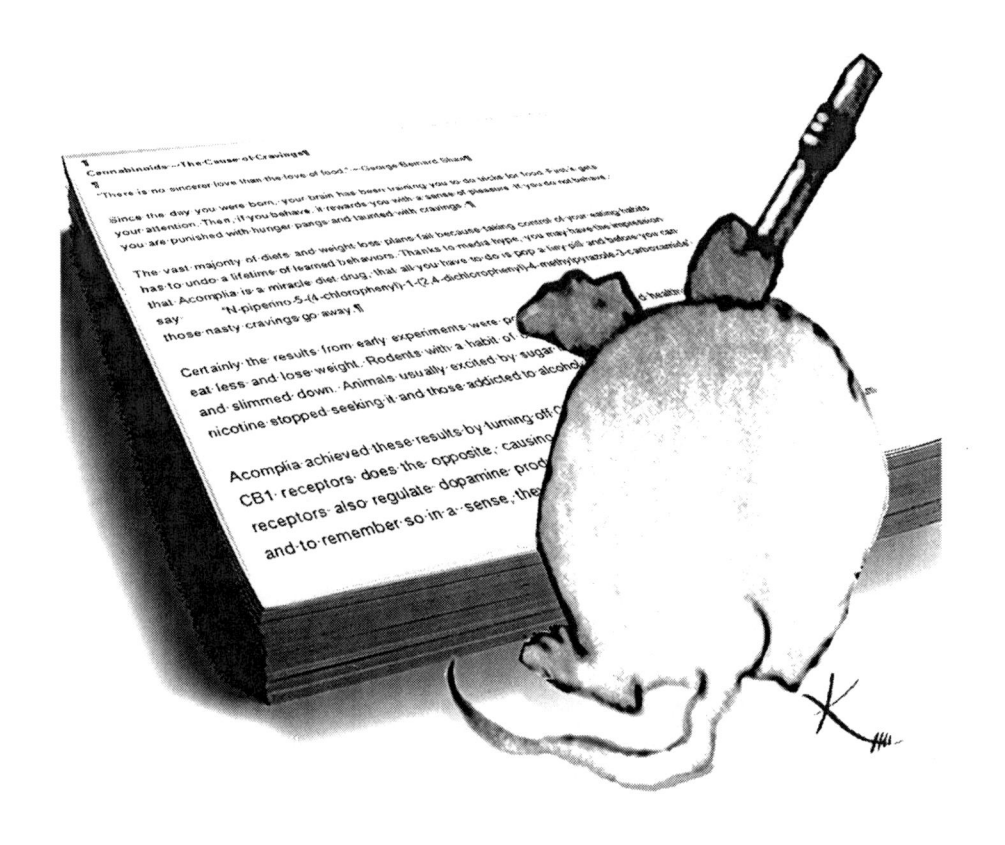

Drugs – No Rodent Left Behind

Your CB1 receptors are part of your brain's reward circuitry. As such, they are a key component of addiction.[107] As we have seen, Acomplia turns of CB1 receptors to reduce cravings for food, alcohol and nicotine - so why not addictive drugs?

Rats have learned to press a lever that infuses heroin directly into their brains until they become firmly addicted. Then, if the amount of heroin is gradually reduced, they can be weaned off the drug until they eventually ignore the lever.

Does this mean that they have kicked the habit? Not really. All it takes is a tiny dose of heroin to make them pump away on the lever as though they had never quit. That's because heroin over-stimulates their opioid receptors and triggers a spurt of dopamine secretion.

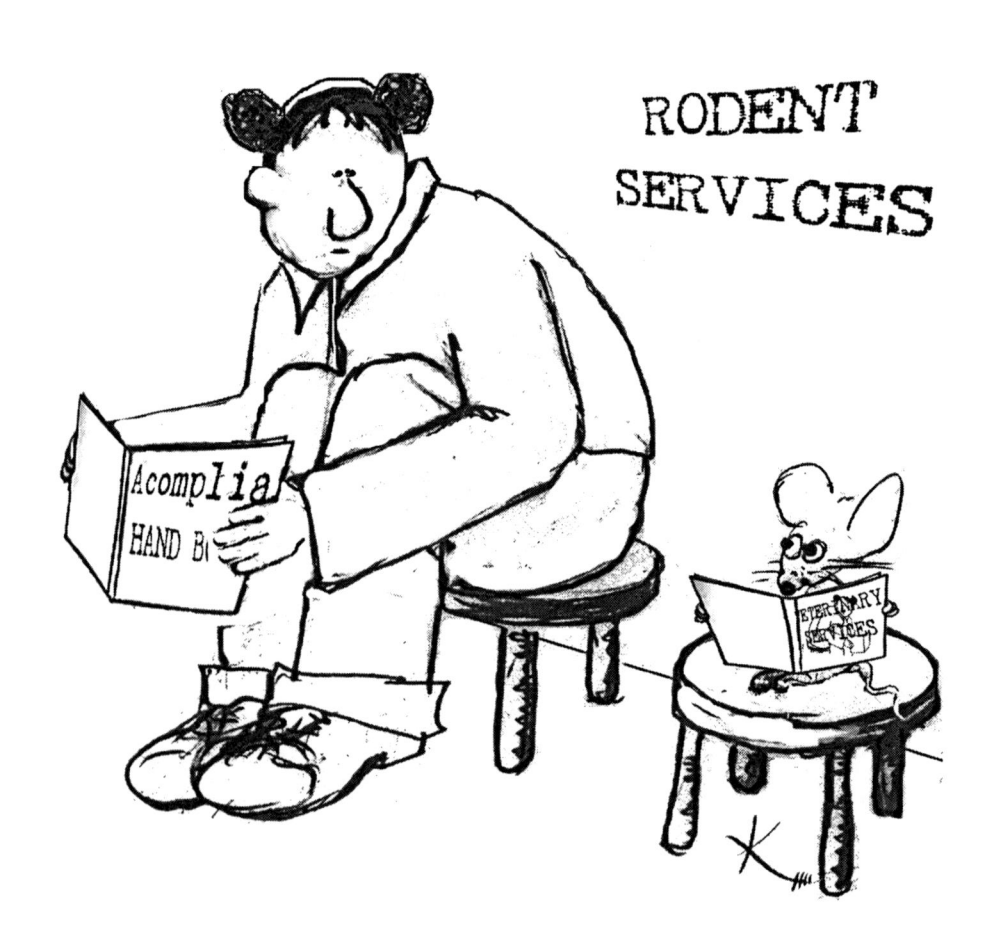

As dopamine floods their brains, it brings a resurgence of pleasurable memories linked to lever pressing. Naturally, you would probably expected a hard drug like heroin to have that effect. Would it surprise you to learn that your own cannabinoids can do exactly the same thing?

Rats who had beaten their addiction to heroin were driven to renewed lever pressing by a single dose of anandamide. Addiction and addictive behavior is fully restored simply by stimulating CB1 receptors.[108]

After taking Acomplia, rats who were free to inject themselves with heroin did so less often. In fact, if Acomplia is put directly into a part of the brain called the cerebellum, they stop lever pressing completely.[109]

The cerebellum is associated with learning and mobility and, in rats, is especially thick with CB1 receptors.[110] Acomplia may reduce cravings to the point that the rats lose interest in heroin or it may suppresses memories sufficiently that the rats forget why the lever is there. Either way, Acomplia is interesting as a possible treatment for heroin addiction.

Cocaine is another matter. Acomplia fails to have any effect on mice addicted to cocaine because it does not work through the CB1 receptors.[111] Instead, it binds to a protein that carries dopamine away and hampers its ability to do its job. As a result, dopamine lingers longer and accumulates in the brain's pleasure centers.[112]

The story of marijuana is quite different. Some lab rats that were addicted to marijuana became so tolerant of the drug that they eventually derived no pleasure from it. Even so, their addiction was so strong that they could not live without it.

Attempting to provide some relief from their cravings, researchers gave them a dose of Acomplia. Sadly, it triggered muscle spasms and life-threatening withdrawal.[113]

Then someone discovered that taking Acomplia before the marijuana prevented intoxication and avoided withdrawal symptoms. That opened the way for experiments on humans.

In 2001, in the first study of its kind, 63 healthy men who regularly smoked marijuana, enrolled in a program to monitor their heart rates and psychological effects to determine if Acomplia could reduce their dependency on the drug.

Typically, marijuana increases the heart rate, but it turned out that Acomplia lowered it by an average of 59%. In addition, nearly half the men said they did not feel intoxicated and none of them complained of serious side effects.[114]

Today, treatment of marijuana addiction in rodents is routine, but there is still no approved treatment for marijuana dependence in humans.[115]

*"I plan on living forever.
So far, so good."*
~ Unknown

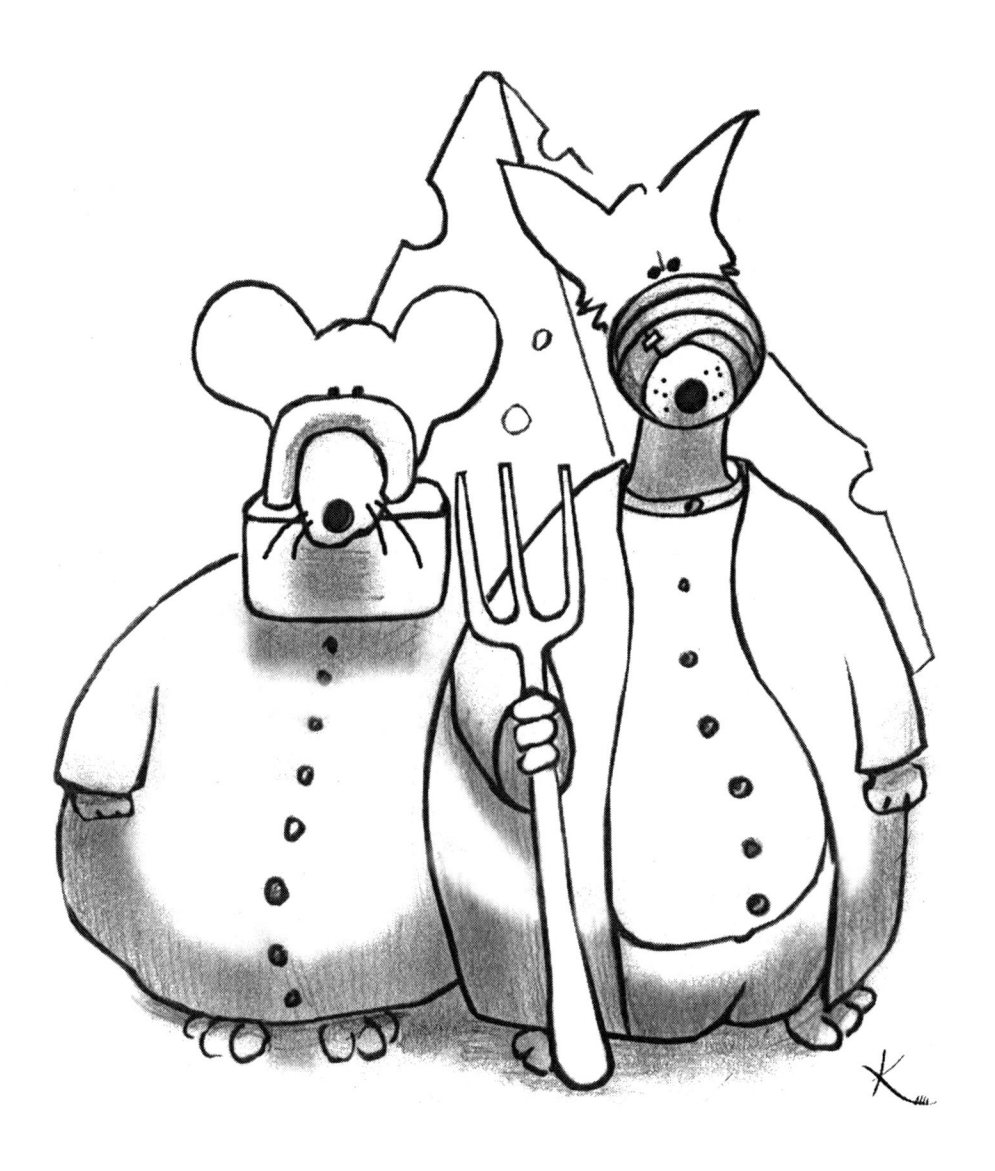

Acomplia - Innovation In Research

Is Acomplia a miracle drug? Perhaps not, but it has unveiled much about cravings and weight loss that was inexplicable only a few short years ago and inspired a rush of innovative research in pursuit of safe and effective weight-loss treatments.

A UK company, Vernalis, has a drug similar to Acomplia in phase 2 trials that helped one patient lose 24 pounds in less than three weeks although the average weight loss was 11 pounds over 16 days on 100 mg.[145] Better yet; the incidence of side effects like nausea and depression was very low.[146]

Merck and Pfizer, two of the world's largest pharmaceutical companies, also have drugs in phase 3 trials that target CB-1 receptors.

Another new weight loss drug still in the experimental stage is a peptide known as TLQP-21. Because peptides break down rapidly, this protein cannot be taken as a pill. It must be injected directly into the brain.[147] Mice undergoing treatment stay slim no matter how fattening their diets are. In theory, it could do the same for humans. If it's all the same, I'll let you try it first.

Oxyntomodulin is another treatment delivered via injection, only this time it goes into your stomach.[148] This hormone occurs naturally in your intestines to suppress appetite, but a booster shot three times a day (before each meal) helped obese patients lose an average of 5 pounds over four weeks.

Nasal Sprays

Obestatin is a newly discovered intestinal hormone that signals the brain to eat less. It acts in opposition to ghrelin, a hormone in the stomach that causes hunger.

Strangely, both hormones are produced by the same gene. That's like having only one pedal in your car for both breaking and accelerating.[149] That aside, obestatin is too fragile to be taken orally and would have to be injected unless it can be delivered as a nasal spray.

PYY is another fragile peptide that could best be delivered by inhalation. It too originates in the intestines and reduces appetite, but if you are over weight you produce only a third as much of it as skinny folk do.

Taking a whiff of PYY before meals has helped heavier men and women cut down their calorie intake by 15%. A few patients reported mild nausea as the only side effect.[150] It might be approved for sale in three or four years.

Gastric Pacemakers

Drugs are not the only weight loss treatments in development. New techniques are being tested regularly. For example, between the extremes of attending military boot camp or undergoing drastic by-pass surgery there is a new device that delivers an electrical pulse to your system to help you lose weight.

It's a gastric pacer, a small, battery driven implant that slides under your skin and is wired up to your gut. It won't actually shock you bolt-upright every time to sit down at the table, but it will stimulate a sense of fullness throughout the day.[151]

Vaccines

How good would it be to see the doctor once a year for a shot to prevent weight gain? Vaccines that reduce dopamine production are already in development to curb cravings and addiction to nicotine. It's early days, but this line of research could one day result in treatments for prevention of several disorders.

False Memories

As for the power of food-related memories, a psychologist has successfully replaced memories that trigger cravings with false memories that trigger avoidance using only the power of suggestion. Students who initially liked strawberry ice cream later claimed to dislike it because of a bad experience as a child.[153]

WHAT'S NEW IN WEIGHT-LOSS DRUGS

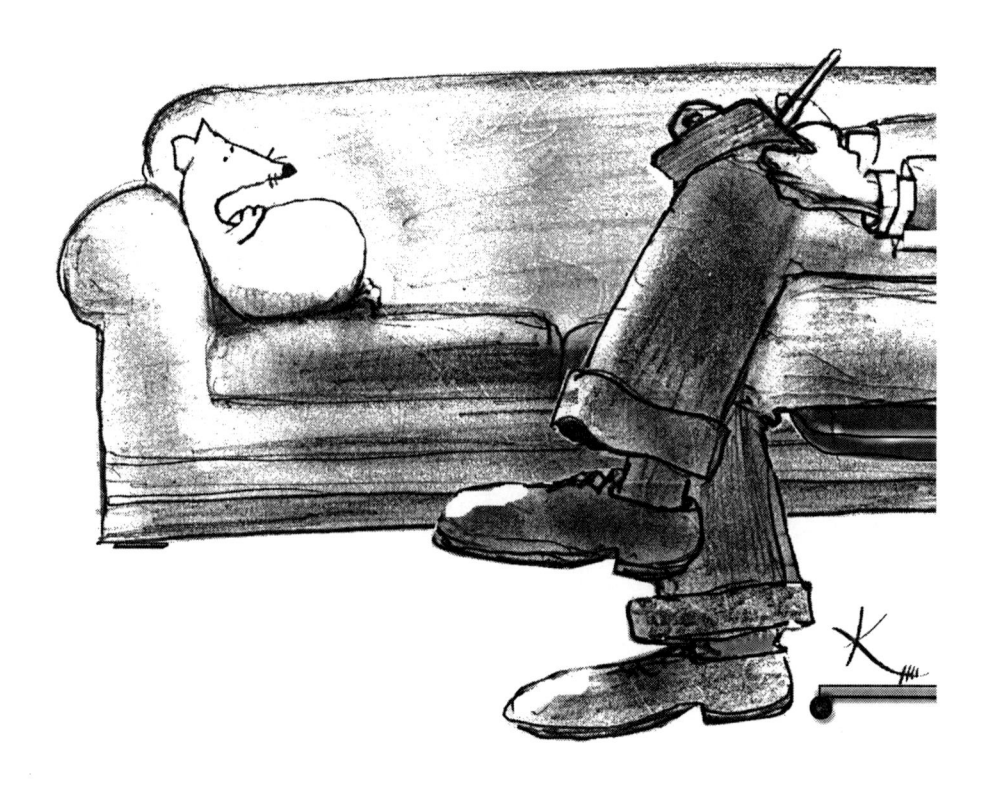

*When your only tool is a hammer,
every problem is a nail.
~ Unknown*

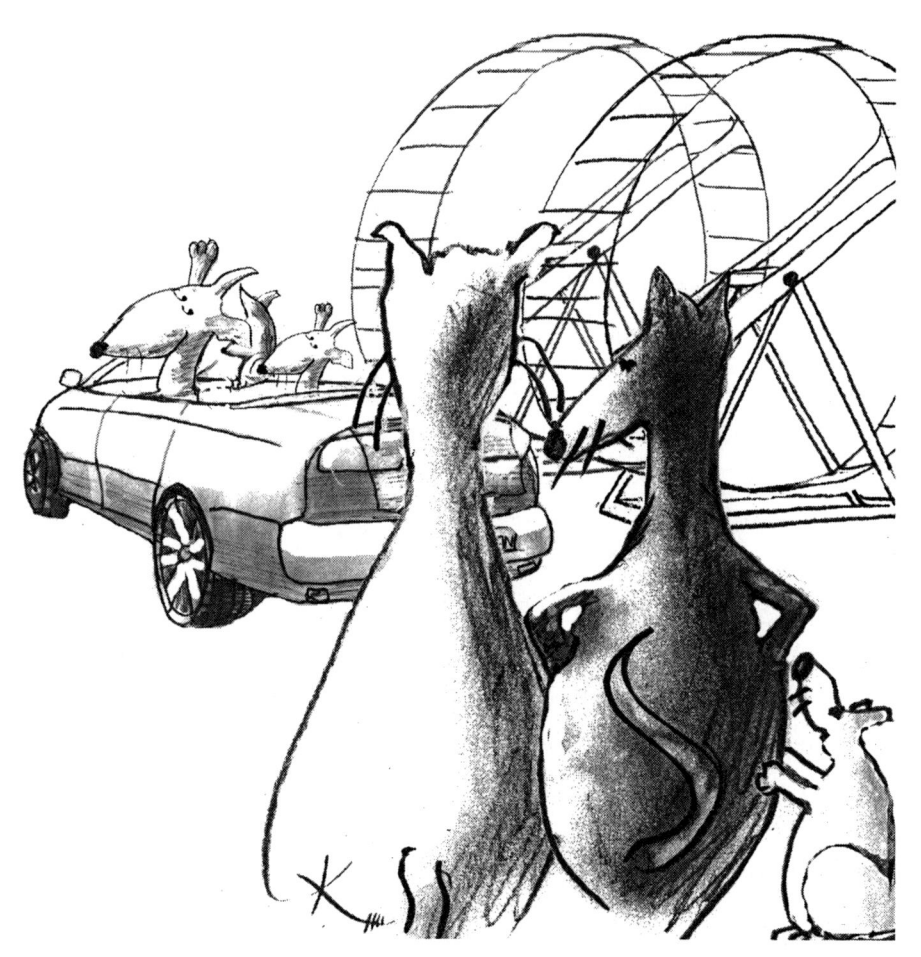

The control group gets new wheels.

Acomplia - Future Treatments

Acomplia has added immensely to our understanding of the human brain. Exposing the role of cannabinoids in food addiction and fat production has moved us closer to unraveling the complex interlocking neural pathways, finely tuned feedback loops and backup systems that complicate research.

We now know that cannabinoids are involved in many overlapping brain systems and that they are linked to a number of medical conditions like diabetes, heart disease, Parkinson's, schizophrenia, anxiety, persistent pain, cancer, memory loss, immune deficiencies and infertility.

Here are some areas of medical research where Acomplia is under investigation as a treatment for illness and behavioral problems; as an antibiotic to protect the immune system; and as a diagnostic tool in disease prevention.

Infertility

Would you have guessed that Acomplia would help human sperm swim faster? It's true. If you put a drop of anandamide on the head of a sperm cell it gets lazy and slows down.[116] If you splash it with a solution of Acomplia it swims away wagging its tail faster than ever.

Prostate Cancer

Cannabinoids regulate cell growth within the prostate gland. If it turns out that they are responsible for the mutation and proliferation of cancerous prostate cells, then Acomplia may have a role to play in the prevention of this leading cause of death among American men.[117]

Pain

In Italy, researchers found that Acomplia relieves the tingling or burning sensations that accompany nerve damage.[118]

This type of pain is often the result of demyelination of nerve fibers, the erosion of protective insulation. Repeated treatments with Acomplia prevent damage and promote healing.

Parkinson's

Rats with advanced Parkinson's disease sometimes benefit from treatment with Acomplia.[119] Parkinson's causes a loss of control over voluntary movement and often leads to tics and spasms called dyskinesia. CB1 receptors influence muscle movement by regulating GABA and other neurotransmitters in the mid-brain, the very place where damaged cells cause dyskinesia.

Currently there is no definitive test for Parkinson's disease. Blood tests, MRI and CT scans help rule out other diseases, but a definitive diagnosis, especially early on, is not possible. Thanks to Acomplia and a growing interest in cannabinoids, that situation may be about to change.

Researchers noticed that monkeys with Parkinson's had high levels of cannabinoids in the mid-brain – from 50% to 90% higher.[120] In the future, monitoring cannabinoid levels could warn of early onset.

Immune System

Acomplia showed some promise as an antibiotic after preventing the spread of Brucellosis, a bacteria that relies on CB1 receptor signaling.

Brucellosis can cause weeks and months of fevers, headaches and severe body pain.[121] You can catch it from other mammals, either by contact or by eating animal products like unpasteurized cheese and milk. Until now, the only cure was daily injections of multiple antibiotics for up to six weeks.

Cannabinoids aid the growth of Brucella bacteria by interfering with the function of macrophages, immune cells that snack on bacteria and dying cells that might contribute to disease.[122] Macrophages get their name from the Greek words *makros* and *phagein*, meaning big eaters.

Acomplia boosts the immune system by increasing the availability of nitric oxide. That's right, macrophages kill foreign bacteria with the same toxic poison emitted by cars and power plants. But nitric oxide is also an important messenger molecule that dilates arteries to increase blood flow and speed macrophages into battle.[123]

What's more, over-active cannabinoids are known to slow down your immune system by interfering with D2 dopamine receptors.[124] By blocking CB1 receptors, Acomplia frustrates those cannabinoids and improves immune response times.

Dopamine Receptors

This all sounds very promising, but the use of Acomplia is not without complications. For instance, in the above case, people with low D2 receptor activity are prone to uncontrolled brain signaling that causes random tics and odd behaviors.

WHAT'S NEW IN WEIGHT-LOSS DRUGS 155

It appears that cannabinoids play a role in preventing such disorders including schizophrenia and Tourette's syndrome.[125] So while Acomplia may enhance your immune system, it might also introduce unwanted symptoms.[126-127]

Cannabinoids are so intricately woven into every aspect of your being that tinkering with them is bound to have some unexpected consequences. We are all wired differently and there is no way to know how Acomplia would affect you personally.

For example, nuclear imaging reveals that people who are shy or awkward in public have D2 receptors that aren't firing on all cylinders.[128] It's conceivable that Acomplia could undermine self confidence and turn a wall flower into a hermit.

Decision Making

As you know by now, dopamine receptors reward and reinforce the important decisions you make in life.[129] They influence your taste in friends and your choice of marriage partner. In theory, if Acomplia reduces your dopamine activity it might change your preferences or even your personality.

Social Awareness

Consider how Acomplia influences the action of one small molecule called oxytocin. Oxytocin is a messenger molecule responsible for your desire to mate. It also invokes parental instincts and promotes breast feeding. You depend on it for orgasm!

Oxytocin receptors are found all over your brain, but they cluster thickly in regions like the amygdala where memories are processed. When oxytocin receptors are blocked, mice suffer from social amnesia. They forget who their partners are and neglect their young.

CB1 receptors are located downstream from oxytocin receptors, so they are in a position to alter oxytocin signaling.[130] We know this is true because oxytocin by itself reduces feeding in mice, but blocking CB1 receptors with Acomplia causes a much stronger effect. Does that mean Acomplia could improve your sex life? Who knows?

Brain Development

This much is certain, CB1 receptors play a delicate role in fetal brain development. After birth, receptors continue to grow and spread in specific areas of the brain for weeks and months.[131] In new born mice, CB1 receptors are at least partially responsible for the suckling reflex.[132]

If you are pregnant or breast feeding, Acomplia could derail your child's brain development. Over-stimulation of CB1 receptors with marijuana in fetal mice causes epileptic seizures. Too little activation, due to Acomplia, leaves them comatose.[133]

Anxiety

As you can see, turning off CB1 receptors is sometimes helpful - sometimes harmful. Perhaps you can now appreciate how difficult it is to make drugs with no side effects.

Take stress, for example. Stress is a product of CB1 receptor signaling.[134] Nightmares, fatigue, dizziness, headaches, neck pain, racing heart and panic attacks are typical symptoms made worse by active CB1 receptors. If you are over-eating as a way to cope with stress, you may be over-activating your cannabinoids and fueling your anxiety.

In a few cases, steady doses of Acomplia have helped to control stress. Results were so promising that Acomplia was considered as a treatment for post-traumatic stress disorder, a severe form of anxiety linked to horrific memories.

Then it turned out that Acomplia sustained *learned fear responses*.[135] In other words, Acomplia had the opposite effect, either making it easier to recall traumatic events and bad memories that are best forgotten or entrenching fearful behavior.

Paradoxically, CB1 knockout mice and mice treated with Acomplia are very resistant to anxiety. But it comes at a price. In the long run, they suffer more brain damage than normal mice.[136-137-138] They live stress-free but significantly shorter lives.

Like mice, you too need cannabinoids to avoid cellular injury due to oxidation, to sustain regular blood supplies to individual cells and to keep your brain from aging too quickly.[139]

Memory

Acomplia has improved memory and learning in some experiments and actually reversed brain damage caused by over-active cannabinoids.[140-141-142-143] Then again, cannabinoids can improve memory too: they assist with mnemonics, a process that organizes information for easy recall. They also help erase unused and obsolete memories to keep your mind sharp and uncluttered.[144]

Obviously there are many reasons not to interfere with your CB1 receptors. With the development of more refined drugs it might be possible to tweak your cannabinoid system rather than turn it off completely. When that time comes, Acomplia may be viewed as a blunt instrument rather than a cutting-edge tool.

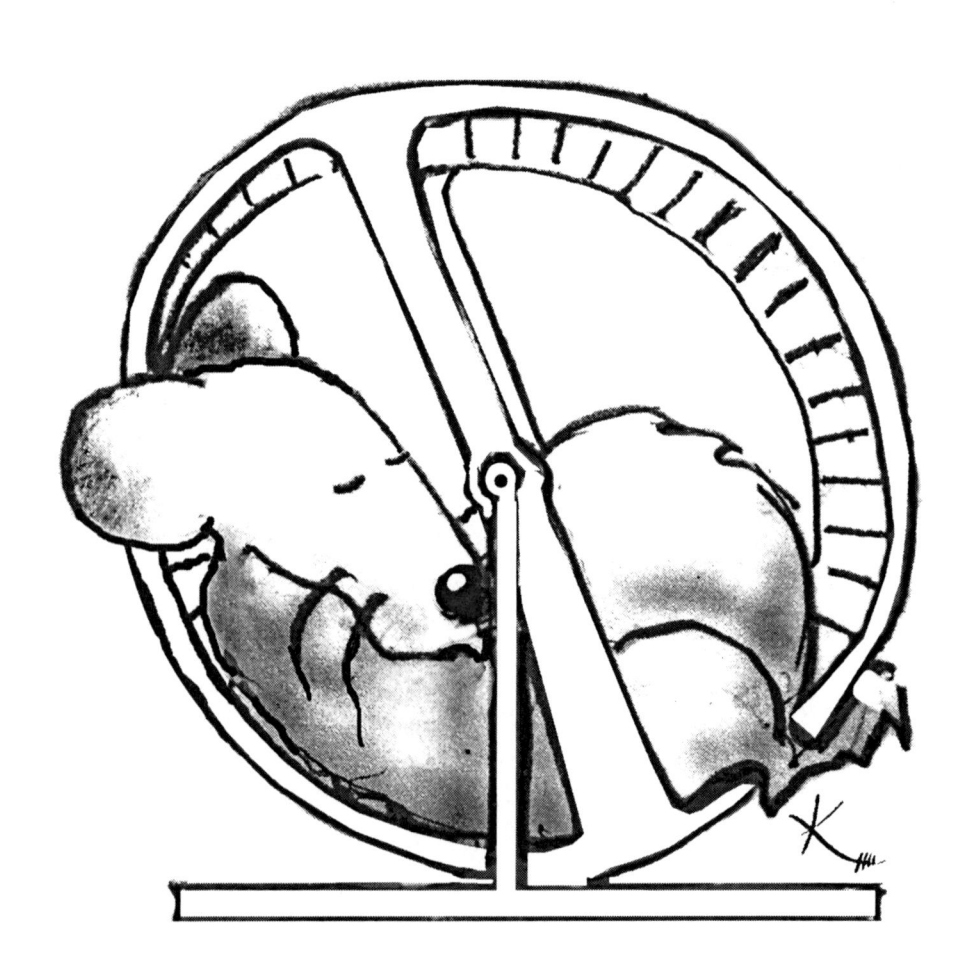

Final Note

In America, where Acomplia still awaits approval, we have an opportunity to see how well Acomplia works. Around the world, tens of thousands of over-weight patients take Acomplia everyday as part of a vast, human experiment. Only time and testing will tell us what we need to know about potential side effects and who is most at risk for them.

The discovery of Acomplia has accelerated brain research and continues to expand our understanding of food, alcohol and nicotine addiction. It has also given medicine important new tools in the battle against obesity, diabetes and heart disease. New prescription drugs and novel therapies are in the pipeline that were unimaginable a few years ago.

Thanks to Acomplia, patients have renewed hope that doctors will soon be able to reduce their cravings, promote fat loss and protect them against weight-related illness.

~

INDEX

2
2AG (2-arachidonyl-glycerol) 64

A
acetylcholine 134-136
Acomplia 5- 7, 10, 11, 13, 15-17, 27, 29, 40, 42, 44, 47, 48, 51-53, 59, 60, 64, 66, 67, 70-72, 77, 78, 82-84, 89-92, 95, 96, 98, 101, 102, 107-111, 113-116, 121, 124, 125, 127, 128, 132-134, 137, 139-141, 145-152, 157
addiction 9, 11, 77, 79, 91, 132, 139-142, 145
adenylate cyclase 65, 66
adiponectin 44, 53
alcohol 40, 64, 77, 79, 121-128, 131, 139
alcoholism 121, 124, 128
Alli 39
American College of Cardiology 137
amygdala 65, 156
amylase 24
anandamide 21, 64, 65, 70-72, 82, 140, 146
Axokine 36

B
binge eating 84
bliss molecule 21, 64, 70
BMI 32, 34
Body Mass Index 33
brain damage 124, 157
Brucellosis 153, 154
Bupropion 136

C
calories 50
cancers 9, 11, 29, 122
cannabinoid receptors, 19, 20, 25-27, 43, 44
cannabinoid system 47, 48, 82, 83, 131, 158
cannabinoids 50, 64-67, 72, 82, 125, 126, 140, 145, 146-149, 151, 152-155, 157
cannabis, 19, 20
caudate 77
CB1 receptors 44-47, 52, 60, 64-67, 69, 124-128, 132, 139-141, 147, 148, 152-158
central nervous system 36, 38, 65, 123
cerebellum 140
cholesterol, 11, 31, 34, 36, 38, 50, 102, 108, 114-116
clinical trials, 89, 90, 96, 97, 109, 136, 146
cocaine, 141
cravings, 11, 24, 39, 47, 53, 60, 64, 66, 75-79, 136, 139, 140, 145, 152, 155

D
depression, 31, 59, 95, 96, 103, 110, 116
diabetes 9, 11, 29, 30, 38, 40, 92, 104, 110, 114-116, 146
dopamine, 36, 58-60, 64, 78, 122, 131-141, 155
dopamine receptors, 148, 154, 155

E
enkephalin, 60
enzyme, 24, 45, 126, 134

F
fat, 10, 17, 20, 25, 30, 31, 36, 38, 40, 44, 49, 52, 103, 114, 145
fatty acids, 40, 44
FDA 36, 37, 38, 90, 96, 109, 114, 136, 137
fenfluramine, 35
Fen-phen 35, 36, 37
forebrain 16, 59, 125

G
GABA 58, 123, 124, 147
gamma-aminobutyric acid 123
gastrointestinal system 52
gene splicing 45
genes 39, 45, 124, 125
genetic mutation 84

globesity 30, 32, 34, 40, 84
glucose 34, 49, 50, 52, 53, 92, 113
glutamate 123
G-protein coupled receptors 66

H
heart 9, 11, 29, 30, 37, 65, 82, 83, 91, 103, 104, 110, 122, 141, 146, 152, 155, 159
heroin 58, 71, 140, 141
hippocampus 65, 78
hormones 10, 17, 25, 58, 60, 83, 125
hunger 10, 16, 17, 19, 20, 25, 36, 44, 47-51, 60-66, 70, 71, 124, 136, 153
hypothalamus 65

I
immune system 82, 146, 148, 149
infertility 146
insula cortex 77
insulin 49, 50, 53, 92, 113-115
International Congress on Obesity 30
International Obesity Task Force 32
intestinal tract 24

K
knockout mouse 45, 46

L
learning 3, 65, 77, 78, 140, 157
leptin 38, 39, 49, 50, 53
ligase 45
limbic system 66
liver 10, 17, 24

M
magnetic resonance imaging 31
marijuana 10, 20, 51, 58, 141, 142, 156
Mayo Clinic 37
MC receptors 84
memories 59, 60, 65, 78, 133, 134, 136, 140, 148, 156, 157, 158
Meridia 38
messenger molecules 16, 17, 123, 125
metabolic syndrome 30, 49, 50, 53, 79, 95, 102, 115
midbrain 44, 59, 125
mood 36, 47, 123, 125

morphine 60, 70, 71, 77
MRI 31, 77, 147
muscle 17, 40, 52, 141, 152

N
naloxone 70, 71, 72, 77
nasal spray 152
National Institute of Health 34
National Institute on Alcohol Abuse and Alcoholism 121, 128
nausea 95, 96, 103, 146, 147
neurons 53
neurotransmitter 123, 134
nicotine 58, 59, 60, 64, 77, 91, 122, 123, 131-136, 139
NicVAX 136
NIH 34
nitric oxide 154
nucleus accumbens 78, 135

O
ob gene 39
obesity 30, 34, 39, 84, 109, 110
Obestatin 153
opioid receptors 21, 60, 70-72, 77, 128, 140
opioids 60, 72
Orlistat 38, 39
oxidation 151
oxyntomodulin 146
oxytocin 155, 156

P
pain 10, 21, 70, 71, 124, 152, 153, 154, 157
pancreas, 24
pandemic 30
parasympathetic nervous system 134
Phentermine 36, 37
phospholipase 126
PLA2 126
placebo 39, 91, 96-98, 102, 103, 108-110, 114-116
Pondimin 36
prefrontal cortex 65
primitive brain 16
protein 21, 141, 146

R
randomized, 96, 103
rationing 46, 50
receptors 15-17, 19, 20, 24, 27, 44, 45, 47, 51, 58, 59, 64, 66, 70, 71, 77, 82, 123-126, 128, 134-136, 139, 140, 141, 146, 153-158
Redux 37
reward 10, 16, 59, 72, 76-78, 135, 139, 155
rimonabant 90
RIO lipids 90
risk 9, 11, 30, 32, 34, 38, 58, 91, 104, 108, 122, 124

S
Sanofi-Aventis 26, 109, 137
schizophrenia 146, 149
Sibutramine 38
side effects 20, 36-39, 47, 70, 95, 96, 98, 102, 109-111, 116, 136, 137, 141, 146, 156, 159
signaling 21, 25, 27, 65, 77, 84, 113, 123, 153-157
sugar 17, 40, 47, 48, 49, 60, 64, 92, 97, 113-116
surgery 31, 147, 154

T
Texas A&M 122
THC 20, 21, 49, 51, 64, 70, 71, 72, 77
TLQP-21 146
Topamax 38
triglycerides 11, 115

V
vaccines 136
Varenicline 136
Vernalis 152

W
Welbutrin 136
will power 72, 135
withdrawal 39, 60, 133-136, 141
World Health Organization (WHO) 30
Wyeth-Ayerst Laboratories 37

X
Xenical 38

REFERENCES

1. Di Marzo V, Matias I; Nat Neurosci. 2005 May
2. Hanus Devane; 1992
3. Rinaldi-Carmona, M, Barth F, Heaulme M, et al.; SR141716A;. FEBS Lett. 1994 Aug
4. U.S. Department of Health & Human Services 2000
5. Paul Zimmet, Chairman: Intern'l Congress on Obesity: Rohan Sullivan in The Toronto Star, Sept 6, 2006
6. National Health and Nutrition Examination Survey (NHANES); 1999-2000
7. Hedley, Allison; CDC National Center for Health Statistics
8. Hellmich, Nanci; USA TODAY 5/2/2005
9. National Health and Nutrition Examination Survey (NHANES); 1999-2000
10. Americans too fat for x-rays; BBC News, Thursday, 27 July 2006
11. National Health and Nutrition Examination Survey (NHANES); 1999-2000
12. Philip James, British Chairman of Inter'l Congress on Obesity: Rohan Sullivan in The Toronto Star, Sept 6, 2006
13. Kate Steinbech, Royal Prince Alfred Hospital, Sydney: Rohan Sullivan in The Toronto Star, Sept 6, 2006
14. http://www.bodybuilders.com/arnold.htm

15. Susan Kelleher & Duff Wilson; The Seattle Times; June 26 - June 30, 2005
16. Susan Kelleher & Duff Wilson; The Seattle Times; June 26 - June 30, 2005
17. Schwartz LM; Woloshin S; Eff Clin Pract. 1999 Mar-Apr;2(2):76-85
18. Drug Discovery Channel: Article; Mar 1 2005 (Vol. 25, No. 5)
19. U.S. Food and Drug Administration; http://www.fda.gov/cder/news/phen/fenphenpr81597.htm
20. U.S. Food and Drug Administration; http://www.fda.gov/bbs/topics/ANSWERS/ANS00835.html
21. Columbia University, Feb. 05; 1999.
22. Paragh G, Bajnok L.; Role of Orlistat in the Treatment of Obesity
23. Bailey,R; About dot com; 07/02/98
24. U.S. Food and Drug Administration (February 7, 2007). FDA Approves Orlistat; 2007-02-07.
25. Schmid, Randolph E; The Washington Post, February 8, 2007. Retrieved on 2007-02-10.
26. Fukuchi S, Hamaguchi K, et al; Exp Biol Med (Maywood). 2004 Jun;229(6):486-93
27. Di Marzo V, Goparaju SK, Wang L, et.al; Nature. 2001 Apr
28. Ward SJ, Dykstra LA; Behav Pharmacol. 2005 Sep;16
29. Simiand J, Keane M, Keane PE, Soubrie P: Behav Pharmacol. 1998
30. Perio A, Barnouin MC, Poncelet M, Soubrie P; Behav Pharmacol. 2001
31. Poireir, Bidouard, Cadrouvele et al; 2005
32. Vickers SP, Webster LJ, Wyatt A, et al; Psychopharmacology (Berl). 2003
33. Carai, Colombo, Gessa; May 10, 2004
34. Mato S, Pazos A, Valdizan EM.1: Eur J Pharmacol. 2002 May 17;443(1-3):43-6
35. Liu YL, Connoley IP, Wilson CA, Stock MJ; Int J Obes (Lond). 2005 Feb
36. Liu YL, Connoley IP, Wilson CA, Stock MJ; Int J Obes (Lond). 2005 Feb

37. Bensaid M, Gary-Bobo M, Esclangon A, et al; Mol Pharmacol. 2003 Apr
38. Gueudet C, Santucci V, Rinaldi-Carmona M, Soubrie P, Le Fur G; Neuroreport. 1995 Jul
39. Duarte C, Alonso R, Bichet N, Cohen C, Soubrie P, Thiebot MH; 1INSERM U.288, 2003 Dec 17
40. BBC; Jan 30, 2003 Fast Food as Addictive as Heroin
41. BBC; Jan 30, 2003 Fast Food as Addictive as Heroin
42. Rinaldi-Carmona M, Le Duigou A, Oustric D, et al; J Pharmacol Exp Ther; 1998
43. Gifford, Andrew; Ashby Charles: Journal of Pharmacology and Experimental Therapeutics; vol.277, No.3, 1996
44. Gifford AN, Bruneus M, Gatley SJ, Lan R, Makriyannis A, Volkow ND; J Pharmacol Exp Ther.1999 Feb
45. Rinaldi-Carmona M, Le Duigou A, Oustric D, et al; J Pharmacol Exp Ther; 1998
46. Gifford AN, Bruneus M, Gatley SJ, Lan R, Makriyannis A, Volkow ND; J Pharmacol Exp Ther.1999 Feb
47. Sim-Selley LJ, Brunk LK, Selley DE; Eur J Pharmacol. 2001 Mar
48. Hsieh C, Brown S, Derleth C, Mackie K; J Neurochem. 1999 Aug
49. Williams CM, Kirkham TC; Psychopharmacology (Berl). 1999 Apr
50. Williams CM, Kirkham TC; Pharmacol Biochem Behav. 2002 Jan-Feb
51. Adams IB, Compton DR, Martin BR; J Pharmacol Exp Ther. 1998 Mar
52. Kirkham TC, Williams CM; Psychopharmacology (Berl). 2001 Jan
53. Rowland NE, Mukherjee M, Robertson K; Psychopharmacology (Berl). 2001 Dec
54. Rowland NE, Mukherjee M, Robertson K; Psychopharmacology (Berl). 2001 Dec
55. Pietras TA, Rowland NE; Eur J Pharmacol. May, 2002
56. Plunkett Research Ltd; Food Industry Overview; 17-Feb-2006.

57. Source: U.S. Census Bureau, Population Division; January 03, 2006
58. Pelchat, Johnson, Chan, Valdez, Raglandc; NeuroImage 23 (2004)
59. Packard MG, Knowlton BJ (2002); Annu Rev Neurosci 25:563-593
60. Bechara, A.; Damasio, A. R.; Damasio H. & Anderson, S.W. (1994); Cognition 50: 7-15.
61. Graybiel AM (2005) The basal ganglia: learning new tricks and loving it. Curr Opin Neurobiol 15:638-644.
62. Nasir H. Naqvi, David Rudrauf, Hanna Damasio, Antoine Bechara. (2007); Science 315 (5811): 531-534. DOI:10.1126/science.1135926.
63. Arne D. Ekstrom, Michael J. Kahana, Jeremy B. Caplan, et al.; Nature, Vol 425; 11 Sept 2003; www.nature.com/nature.
64. Olds J, Milner P (1954); J Comp Physiol Psychol 47 (6): 419-27
65. Verty AN, Singh ME, McGregor IS, Mallet PE: Psychopharmacology (Berl). 2003 Jul
66. Wagner JA, Hu K, Bauersachs J, et al;. J Am Coll Cardiol. 2001 Dec;38(7):2048-54.
67. Wagner JA, Varga K, Kunos G; J Mol Med. 1998 Nov-Dec;76(12):824-36.
68. Wagner JA, Varga K, Ellis EF, et al; Nature. 1997 Dec 4; 390(6659):518-21
69. Cainazzo MM, Ferrazza G, Mioni C, et al; Eur J Pharmacol. 2002 Apr 19;441(1-2):91-7.Verty 04
70. Varga K, Wagner JA, Bridgen DT, Kunos G; FASEB J. 1998 Aug;12(11):1035-44.
71. Cainazzo MM, Ferrazza G, Mioni C, et al; Eur J Pharmacol. 2002 Apr 19;441(1-2):91-7.Verty 04
72. Lubrano-Berthelier C, Dubern B, Lacorte JM, et al; J Clin Endocrinol Metab. 2006 Feb 28;
73. Balthasar N, Dalgaard LT, Lee CE, et al; Cell. 2005 Nov 4
74. Verty AN, McFarlane JR, McGregor IS, Mallet PE; Endocrinology. 2004 Jul

75. Pi-Sunyer FX, Aronne LJ, Heshmati HM, Devin J, Rosenstock J; RIO-North America Study Group
76. Boyd, Fremming - March 8, 2005
77. Boyd, Fremming - March 8, 2005
78. Pi-Sunyer FX, Aronne LJ, Heshmati HM, Devin J, Rosenstock J; RIO-North America Study Group
79. Marcio C. Mancini and Alfredo Halpern; Pharmacological Treatment of Obesity; 2006
80. F Xavier Pi-Sunyer, Louis J Aronne, Hassan M Heshmati,et. al; Am J Clin Nutr. 2006 Apr ;83:809-16
81. Scheen AJ; Finer N; Hollander P; Jensen MD; Van Gaal LFP: Lancet. 2006 Nov 11;368(9548):1660-72
82. WHO, Global Status Report on Alconol 2004
83. Chen, Wei-Jung; Alcoholism; Texas A&M Health Science Centre; Star, Wed. July 26, 2006
84. Heinz, Andreas; Scientific American MIND magazine, April/May 2006
85. Basavarajappa, Hungund; Oct 1, 2004
86. Wang L, Liu J, Harvey-White J, Zimmer A, Kunos G; Proc Natl Acad Sci U S A;. Feb, 2003
87. Colombo G, Vacca G, Serra S, Carai MA, Gessa GL; Eur J Pharmacol, 2004 Sep
88. Lallemand F, Soubrie P, De Witte P; Alcohol, 2004 Nov-Dec
89. Basavarajappa, Hungund; Oct 1, 2004
90. Basavarajappa, Hungund; Oct 1, 2004
91. McGregor IS, Gallate JE;Addict Behav. 2004 Sep
92. Gallate JE, McGregor IS; Psychopharmacology (Berl). 1999 Mar
93. Colombo G, Vacca G, Serra S, Carai MA, Gessa GL. Eur J Pharmacol. 2004 Sep
94. Vacca G, Serra S, Brunetti G, Carai MA, Gessa GL, Colombo G; Eur J Pharmacol. Jun, 2002
95. Gessa, Serra, Vacca, Carai, Colombo; Alcohol Alcohol. 2005 Jan-Feb;40(1):46-53. Epub 2004 Dec 6. PMID: 15582988

96. Warren G Magnuson Clinical Center (CC)Sponsored by: National Institute on Alcohol Abuse and Alcoholism (NIAAA)
97. Ducobu J. - Service de Medecine, CHU Tivoli, La Louviere, ULB Rev Med Brux;2005 May-Jun;26(3):159-64
98. Le Foll, Goldberg; July 12, 2004
99. Forget B, Hamon M, Thiebot MH; Psychopharmacology (Berl). 2005 Oct;18

100. Cohen C, Perrault G, Griebel G, Soubrie P; Neuropsychophar macology. 2005 Jan
101. Henningfield JE, Fant RV, Buchhalter AR, Stitzer ML;CA Cancer J Clin. 2005 Sep-Oct (not in PubMed)
102. Wiley JL, Lavecchia KL, Martin BR, Damaj MI; Virginia Commonwealth University, Richmond
103. Durcan MJ, Deener G, White J, Johnston JA,et al; GlaxoSmithKline
104. Coe JW, Brooks PR, Vetelino MG, et al; J Med Chem; 2005May19;48(10):3474-7
105. Fagerstrom K, Balfour DJ; Expert Opin Investig Drugs. 2006 Feb;15(2):107-16
106. Dr Anthenelli, American College of Cardiology; March 2004
107. Le Foll, Goldberg; Oct 27, 2004
108. Fattore L, Spano S, Cossu G, Deiana S, Fadda P, Fratta W; Neuropharmacology. 2005 Jun
109. Navarro M, Carrera MR, Del Arco I, et al; Eur J Pharmacol. 2004 Oct
110. Casu MA, Pisu C, Sanna A, Tambaro S, Spada GP, Mongeau R, Pani L.; Brain Res. 2005 Jun 28
111. Lesscher, Hoogveld, Burbach, Ree, Gerrits; April 6, 2004
112. Kilty, J. E., Lorang, D. & Amara, S. G; Science (New York, N. Y.) 254, 578-579 (1991).
113. Tsou K, Patrick SL, Walker JM; Eur J Pharmacol. 1995 Jul 14
114. Huestis MA, Gorelick DA, Heishman SJ, et al; Arch Gen Psychiatry. 2001 Apr
115. Hart C.L; Drug Alcohol Depend. 2005 Nov
116. Rossato M, Ion Popa F, Ferigo M, Clari G, Foresta C; J Clin Endocrinol Metab. 2005 Feb

117. Sanchez MG, Sanchez AM, Ruiz-Llorente L, Diaz-Laviada I; Alcala University, Madrid, Spain.
118. Costa B, Trovato AE, Colleoni M, Giagnoni G, Zarini E, Croci T; Pain. 2005 Jul;11
119. Fernandez-Espejo E, Caraballo I, de Fonseca FR, et. al; 2005 Apr
120. van der Stelt M, Fox SH, Hill M, Crossman AR, Petrosino S, Di Marzo V, Brotchie; JM FASEB J. 2005 Jul
121. CDC.gov; Coordinating Center for Infectious Diseases; Division of Bacterial and Mycotic Diseases; October 6, 2005
122. Gross A, Terraza A, Marchant J, Bouaboula M, et.al; J Leukoc Biol. 2000 Mar
123. Waksman Y, Olson JM, Carlisle SJ, Cabral GA; J Pharmacol Exp Ther. 1999 Mar
124. Alonso R, Voutsinos B, Fournier M, Labie C, et.al; Neuroscience, 1999
125. Ferrer B, Gorriti MA, Palomino A, Gornemann I, et al; Eur J Pharmacol. 2007 Mar 22;559(2-3):180-3
126. Meltzer HY, Arvanitis L, Bauer D, Rein W; Meta-Trial Study Group; Am J Psychiatry. 2004 Jun;161(6):975-84
127. Poncelet M, Barnouin MC, Breliere JC, Le Fur G, Soubrie P; Psychopharmacology (Berl). 1999 May
128. Schneier et al 2000
129. Young, Larry J: The Neurobiology of Social Recognition, Approach, and Avoidance; Dept. of Psychiatry, Center for Behavioral Neuroscience, Emory University, Atlanta, GA
130. Verty, McFarlane, McGregor, Mallet; June 3, 2004
131. Romero J, Garcia-Palomero E, Berrendero F, Garcia-Gil L, Hernandez ML, Ramos JA,
132. Fernandez-Ruiz JJ; Synapse. 1997 Jul;26(3):317-23
133. Fride E, Foox A, Rosenberg E,et. al; Eur J Pharmacol. 2003 Feb 7;461(1):27-34.
134. Bernard C, Milh M, Morozov YM, Ben-Ari Y, Freund TF, Gozlan H; Proc Natl Acad Sci U S A. 2005 Jun 28
135. Chatwal JP, Davis M, Maguschak KA, Ressler KJ; Neuropsychopharmacology. 2005 Mar

136. Varvel SA, Anum EA, Lichtman AH; Psychopharmacology (Berl). 2005 Jun
137. Griebel G, Stemmelin J, Scatton B; Biol Psychiatry. 2005 Feb
138. Degroot A, Nomikos GG; Eur J Neurosci. 2004 Aug
139. Kim SH, Won SJ, Mao XO, Jin K, Greenberg DA; J Pharmacol Exp Ther. 2005 Apr
140. Kim SH, Won SJ, Mao XO, Jin K, Greenberg DA; J Pharmacol Exp Ther. 2005 Apr
141. Delatte MS, Winsauer PJ, Moerschbaecher JM; Pharmacol Biochem Behav. 2002 Dec
142. Nakamura-Palacios EM, Winsauer PJ, Moerschbaecher JM; Behav Pharmacol. 2000 Aug
143. Brodkin J, Moerschbaecher JM; J Pharmacol Exp Ther. 1997 Sep
144. Mallet PE, Beninger RJ; Psychopharmacology (Berl). Nov 98
145. Varvel SA, Anum EA, Lichtman AH; Psychopharmacology (Berl). 2005 Jun
146. http://www.fiercebiotech.com/press-releases/press-release-vernalis-announces-striking-weight-loss-phase-i-study-v24343-overweight
147. E.J. Mundell; HealthDay Reporter; Anti-Fat Protein Keeps Overeating Mice Slim:
148. Katie Wynne, Adrian J. Park, Caroline J. Small, et al; Diabetes 54:2390-2395, 2005
149. Denise Grady; Hormone Reduced Appetite in Mice: November 11, 2005: http://www.nytimes.com/2005/11/11/health/11hunger.html?_r=1&oref=slogin
150. http://investor.nastech.com/phoenix/
151. Transneuronix Gastric Pacemaker News Release; http://salesandmarketingnetwork.com/news_release.php?ID=2003093: February 1, 2005
152. Dr. Maciej Buchowski; Presentation to the European Congress on Obesity, June 2005
153. Rosie Mestel; Los Angeles Times, Tuesday, August 2, 2005

WHAT'S NEW IN WEIGHT-LOSS DRUGS

The Authors

Kim Walker is a writer, researcher and illustrator; a webmaster for health related web sites; and a constant student of human behavior.

Michael G. Walker teaches molecular biology and medical statistics at Stanford University's School of Medicine. He is also a biotech consultant with numerous publications and patents to his credit.

Together, they reveal the latest discoveries in brain research and molecular biology in a series of popular books that everyone can read and enjoy.

Printed in the United States
108943LV00011B/4-33/P